The Marshall Cavendish Illustrated Encyclopedia of

FAMILY HEALTH

Volume 1

DOCTOR'S ANSWERS

Marshall Cavendish · London, Sydney & New York

Editors Edward Horton
Felicity Smart

Deputy Editor Elizabeth Longley

Senior Sub-Editors Anna Bradley
Sheila Brull
Arlene Sobel

Sub-Editors Jon Kirkwood
Jenny Mohammadi
Alice Peebles
Alan Ross
Raj Sacranie

Editorial Secretary Lynn Smail

Art Editors Maggie Howells
Keith Vollans

Picture Researchers Julia Calloway
Elizabeth Strachan
Vickie Walters

Designers Pamela Alvares
Shirin Patel
Chris Rathbone
Jervis Tuttle
Ginger Wetherley

Artwork Researcher Sally Walters

Picture Stylists Georgina Barker
Ann Kelly
Kiki Lewis

Production Controllers Sue Fuller
Steve Roberts
Roberta Tarran

Production Executive Barry Roberts

Project Executive Robert Paulley

American Consultant P. E. Geraghty M.D. F.C.A.P.

Dr. Trevor Weston Chief Editorial Consultant Dr. Weston
is the Founder and
Chairman of Health Education Audio-Visual
and Consultant Medical Editor of the British
Medical Association's
Family Doctor Publications Unit
and has been both a general practitioner
and hospital consultant.

ISBN 0-86307-127-9 (Set)
ISBN 0-86307-128-7 (Vol 1)

Reference Edition Published 1984
© Marshall Cavendish Limited MCMLXXXI,
MCMLXXXII, MCMLXXXIII

Manufactured in Italy by L.E.G.O. S.p.a. Vicenza

Published by Marshall Cavendish House
58 Old Compton Street
London W1V 5PA

Library of Congress Cataloging in Publication Data
Main entry under title:
Illustrated Encyclopedia of Family Health.

Includes index.
1. Medicine, Popular–Dictionaries. I. Horton,
Edward. II. Smart, Felicity. III. Weston, Trevor.
IV. Title: Family Health. V. Title: Doctor's Answers.
[DNLM: 1. Medicine–Encyclopedias–popular works.
WB 13 129]
RC81. A214 1984 613'.03'21 84-9730
ISBN 0-86307-127-9 (Set)

Cataloging in Publication Data
The Illustrated Encyclopedia of Family Health
1. Family – Health and Hygiene
1. Weston, Trevor
613 RA418.5.F3

Introduction

Our health is our most precious asset — and the health of our families is quite properly a major concern. The *Illustrated Encyclopedia of Family Health* has been specially prepared to fill a unique role in this most crucial area. It is a complete and authoritative guide to your family's health, prepared by a team of experts but written in language that is clear, untechnical and straight to the point.

In every volume you will find the answers to the sort of questions you are most likely to ask, so it's really like having your own family doctor permanently on call. Not, of course, that the *Illustrated Encyclopedia of Family Health* is in any sense a substitute for the enormous range of services provided by the medical profession. But doctors tell us that knowledge is the key to preventing ill health — knowledge of how our body works, knowledge of what we should and should not do to keep it in the best possible working order, and, perhaps most important of all, the knowledge

that enables us to recognise any illness or disorder in its earliest stages, when medical treatment stands the greatest chance of success.

In more than 900 individual articles, arranged alphabetically for easy reference, our experts give you the inside information — dispelling myths and fallacies and replacing them with hard facts, the facts you need at your fingertips to cope with everyday health care. Each article features a special section giving the "Doctor's" straightforward answers to the most relevant questions. Each article is fully illustrated in colour with photographs, informative diagrams and charts, to help in getting the subject across quickly, accurately, and above all, in a manner that is easily understood.

A fully cross-referenced index, an extensive glossary of medical terms and quick reference first-aid handbook can be found in Volume 24 to help you get the most from this valuable work.

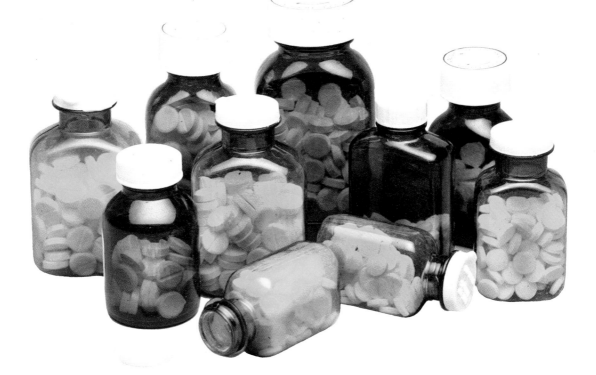

This comprehensive contents list covers, topic by topic, all those subjects included in this 24 volume set.

PREGNANCY & CHILDBIRTH

Abortion
Amniocentesis
Antenatal care
Artificial insemination
Birth
Birthmarks
Blue baby
Bottle feeding
Breast feeding
Breech birth
Caesarean birth
Cleft palate
Club foot
Conception
Congenital disorders
Cystic fibrosis
Eclampsia
Ectopic pregnancy
Episiotomy
Fatherhood
Foetus
Fontanelles
Genetics
German measles
Gynaecology
Hammer toe
Heredity
Inbreeding
Incubators
Induction
Infertility
Lochia
Lordosis
Mastitis
Meconium
Midwifery
Miscarriage
Morning sickness
Motherhood
Multiple birth
Muscular dystrophy
Mutation
Natural childbirth
Navel
Newborn baby
Nursery
Obstetrics
Oedema
Ovaries
Paediatrics
Patent ductus arteriosus
Phantom pregnancy
Phenylketonuria
Pica
Piles

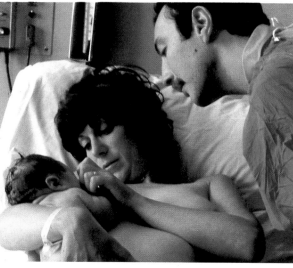

Placenta
Post partum
    haemorrhage
Post-natal depression
Pregnancy
Premature babies
Rhesus factor
Siamese twins
Spina bifida
Still births
Stretch marks
Teratogenesis
Test tube babies
Ultrasound

THE SPECIAL PROBLEMS OF AGE

Ageing
Arthritis
Bedsores
Bunions
Cataracts
Coronary thrombosis
Deafness
Death
Dementia
Diverticulitis
Emphysema
Falls
Gall stones
Geriatrics
Glaucoma
Hearing aids
Hemiplegia

Home helps
Home nursing
Home visits
Hormone replacement
    therapy
Hot flushes
Hydrotherapy
Hypothermia
Incontinence
Institutional care
Invalids
Ischaemia
Kyphosis
Life expectancy
Liver spots
Loneliness
Longevity
Ménière's disease
Menopause
Middle age
Motor neuron disease
Myeloma
Nursing homes
Old age
Osteoarthritis
Osteoporosis
Paget's disease
Parkinson's disease
Phlebitis
Prostate gland
Polycythaemia
Purpura
Rejuvenation
Retirement
Senility
Widowhood
Wrinkles

SPECIAL HEALTH PROBLEMS OF MEN

Baldness
Circumcision
Colour blindness
Erection & ejaculation
Fatherhood
Haemophilia
Impotence
Infertility
Male menopause
Penis
Prostate gland
Reiter's disease
Sperm
Sterilization
Testes
Vasectomy
Widowhood

SPECIAL HEALTH PROBLEMS OF WOMEN

Abortion
Antenatal care
Birth
Breast feeding
Breech birth
Caesarean birth
Cervix and cervical
    smears
Conception
Cosmetics
Cystitis
Depilatories
Dilation & curettage
Eclampsia
Ectopic pregnancy
Episiotomy
Fibroids
Foetus
Gynaecology
Hormone replacement
    therapy
Hot flushes
Hymen
Hysterectomy
Induction
Infertility
Internal examination
Laparoscopy
Lesbianism
Leucorrhoea

Lochia
Masectomy
Mastitis
Menarche
Menopause
Menstruation
Miscarriage
Morning sickness
Motherhood
Natural childbirth
Oestrogen
Oral conception
Ovaries
Pessaries
Phobias
Placenta
Post-natal depression
Post-partum
   haemorrhage
Pregnancy
Pre-menstrual tension
Rape
Salpingitis
Sanitary protection
Slimming
Smear test
Sterilization
Stretch marks
Teratogenesis
Thrush
Toxic shock syndrome
Ultrasound
Uterus
Vagina
Varicose veins
Virginity
Vulva
Widowhood

ALTERNATIVE MEDICINE
Acupuncture
Biofeedback
Eugenics
Euthanasia
Faith healing
Herbalism
Homoeopathy
Humidifiers
Hydrotherapy
Hypnosis
Macrobiotics
Meditation
Naturopathy
Osteopathy
Physiotherapy
Positive health
Preventive medicine
Vegetarianism
Yoga

KEEPING FIT
Antenatal care

Back & backache
Biological clock
Exercise
Health farms
Isometrics
Jet lag
Jogging
Keeping fit
Leisure
Manipulation
Massage
Obesity
Physical fitness
Physiotherapy
Posture
Relaxation
Submersion
Yoga
Zest

PERSONAL HYGIENE
Antiperspirants
Bacteria
Bathing
Bed bugs
Body odour
Cosmetics
Dandruff
Deodorants
Depilatories
Faeces
Fleas
Gargles
Hair care
Halitosis
Health education
Hydatid disease
Hygiene
Insects

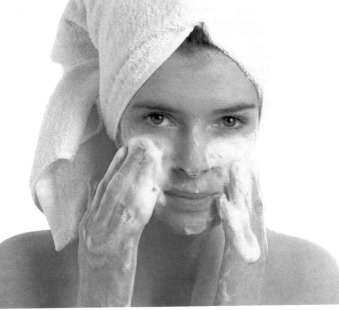

Lice
Nails
Nits
Parasites
Peroxide
Perspiration
Pets
Pimples
Pyorrhoea & gingivitis
Sanitary protection
Scabies
Septic conditions
Smoking
Talcum powder
Toilet training
Verruca
Wax in the ear
Worms

EYES & EYE CARE
Astigmatism
Black eye
Blindness & Braille
Cataracts
Colour blindness
Conjunctivitis
Contact lenses
Cornea
Double vision
Eyes & eyesight
Glaucoma
Keratitis
Lazy eye
Lighting
Night blindness
Nystagmus
Ophthalmology
Optician
Optic nerve
Papilloedema

Retrolental fibroplasia
Spectacles
Squint
Stye
Tunnel vision

INFANCY & CHILDHOOD
Acne
Adenoids
Adolescence
Asthma
Attachment in infancy
Autism
Baby battering
Breath–holding
Burping
Chickenpox
Child development
Comfort habits
Cot death
Crying
Dummies
Disturbed children
Dyslexia
Eczema
Fantasy in childhood
Feeding problems
Fluoride
German measles
Gigantism
Growing pains
Growth
Habits
Handedness
Handicaps
Head banging
Hyperactivity
Imagination
Imitation
Immunization
Incontinence
Incubation
Infancy
Intestines : children's
   disorders
Lazy eye
Learning
Lying
Measles
Mantoux test
Measles
Megacolon
Menarche
Mentally handicapped
   children
Mongolism
Mumps
Murmurs of the heart
Night fears
Nursery
Only child
Paediatrics
Pica

Pigeon chest
Pigeon toes
Pimples
Play
Precocious child
Projectile vomiting
Puberty
Stammering & stuttering
Stealing
Table manners
Tantrums
Teasing
Teeth & teething
Thumb sucking
Toilet training
Toys
Truancy
Twins
Vaccinations
Weaning
Whooping cough

FOOD & DIET
A–vitamin
Appetite
B–vitamins
C–vitamin
Calcium
Cholesterol
D–vitamin
Diet
E–vitamin
Fats
Feeding problems
Food additives
Ginseng
Glucose
Health foods
Iodine
Iron
K–vitamin
Liquid diet
Macrobiotics
Magnesium
Malnutrition
Malt

Milk
Minerals
Monosodium glutamate
Nutrition
Obesity
Potassium
Protein
Salt
Slimming
Starch
Starvation
Sugars
Tea & coffee
Trace elements
Underweight
Vegetarianism
Vitamins
Water

SKIN CARE
Abrasions & cuts
Acne
Ageing
Allergies
Athlete's foot
Bathing
Bed sores
Bites & stings
Blisters
Blushing
Boils
Bruises
Burns
Chafing
Chickenpox
Chilblains
Cold sores
Corns
Cradle cap
Dandruff
Depilatories
Dermatitis
Dressings
Eczema
Grafting
Herpes

Hives
Hypersensitivity
Ichthyosis
Impetigo
Irritants
Itches
Keloids
Keratin
Lacerations
Lice
Lichen
Lipoma
Melanin
Methylated spirit
Mites
Moles
Nettle sting
Nits
Ointments
Peroxide
pH
Photosensitivity
Pimples
Pityriasis rosea
Prickly heat
Pruritus
Psoriasis
Purpura
Rashes
Ringworm
Scabies
Scalding
Scalp
Scars
Sebaceous glands
Shingles
Skin & skin diseases
Sores
Sunburn
Talcum powder
Tattooing
Trichology
Vitiligo
Warts
Whitlow
Wounds
Wrinkles

SEXUAL HEALTH
Abortion
AIDS
Artificial insemination
Circumcision
Contraception
Erection & ejaculation
Genitals
Gonorrhoea
Hermaphrodites
Herpes
Homosexuality
Hormone replacement
  therapy
Impotence
Inbreeding
Incest
Infertility
Intercourse
Lesbianism
Leucorrhoea
Libido
Masturbation
Non–specific urethritis
Oestrogen
Oral contraception
Orgasm
Penis
Rhythm method
Sex
Sex change
Sex education
Sperm
Sterilization
Sublimation
Syphilis
Testes
Test tube babies
Vagina
Vasectomy
Venereal diseases
Virginity
Vulva

ACCIDENTS, EMERGENCIES & FIRST AID
Abrasions & cuts
Accident prevention
Artificial respiration
Bandages
Bites & stings
Black eye
Blackouts
Bleeding
Blisters
Bruises
Burns
Cardiac massage
Choking
Convulsions
Diarrhoea

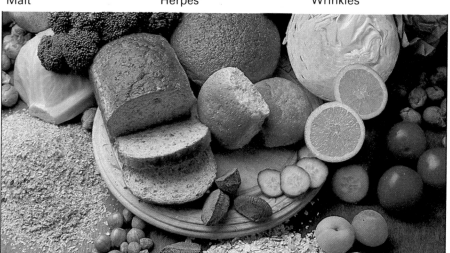

Dislocation
Dog bites
Dressings
Drowning
Electric shock
Emergencies
Emetics
Enteritis
Epilepsy
Exposure
Fainting
Falls
Food poisoning
Fractures
Frost-bite
Gargles
Gas safety
Haemorrhage
Hamstring injuries
Hangover
Head & head injuries
Headache
Heart attack
Heat & heat disorders
Hiccups
Holiday health
Hypoxia
Hysteria
Ice and cold compresses
Indigestion
Injuries
Irritants
Lacerations
Lightning accidents
Mallet finger
Methylated spirits
Mountain sickness
Mushroom poisoning
Nausea
Nettle sting
Numbness
Obstructions
Occupational hazards
Ointments
Overbreathing
Overdoses
Pain killers
Palpitations
Pesticides
Plasters
Poisoning
Proprietary medicines
Pulled muscles
Pulse
Rape
Resuscitation
Road accidents
Scalding
Shock
Smelling salts
Snake–bite
Splinter
Sports medicine
Sprains
Stiffness
Stitch

Strains
Strangulation
Stretchers
Suffocation
Sunburn
Sunstroke
Swallowed objects
Syncope
Temperature
Tetanus
Tourniquet
Travel sickness
Unconsciousness
Vomiting
Whiplash injury
Wounds

WONDERS OF MODERN MEDICINE

Amniocentesis
Anaesthetics
Artificial insemination
Artificial limbs
Biopsy
Blood donor
Blood transfusion
Brain surgery
Caesarean birth
Callipers & braces
Cervix & cervical smears
Colostomy
Contact lenses
Dilation & curettage
Donors
Drip
Electrocardiogram
Electroencephalogram
Endoscopy
Episiotomy
Freezing
Grafting
Gynaecology
Heart transplant
Hydrotherapy
Hysterectomy
Indentification
Incubators
Induction
Injections
Intensive care units
Interferon
Kidney machines
Kidney transplants
Laminectomy
Laparoscopy
Laparotomy
Lasers
Leucotomy
Lithotomy
Local anaesthetics
Lumbar puncture
Mantoux test
Marrow and transplants

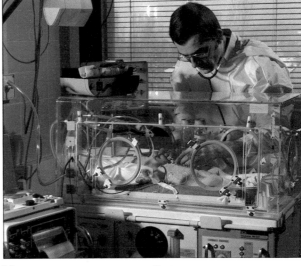

Mastectomy
Medical research
Medical technology
Medicines
Microbiology
Microsurgery
Monitoring equipment
Nephrectomy
Neurology & neurosurgery
Nursing
Obstetrics
Open heart surgery
Operating theatre
Ophthalmology
Optician
Organ removal
Orthodontics
Orthopaedics
Osteopathy
Oxygen
Pacemaker
Paediatrics
Pathology
Pharmacy
Physiotherapy
Plastic surgery
Post-operative care
Premedication
Prostheses
Public health
Radiotherapy
Respirators
Resuscitation
Screening
Sex change
Smear test
Speculum
Sphygmomanometer
Splints
Sterilization
Steroids
Stethoscope
Stoma care
Stomach pump
Surgery

Sutures
Syringeing
Test tube babies
Thermography
Tracheotomy
Transplants
Vaccinations
Vagotomy
Vasectomy
Ventricular fibrillation
Veterinary medicine
X–rays

MEDICINES & DRUGS

Amphetamines
Anabolic steroids
Anaesthetic
Antibiotics
Aspirin & analgesics
Barbiturates
Barium meal
Cannabis
Diuretics
Drip
Drug abuse
Emetics
Enema
Expectorants
Fluoride
Gargles
Herbalism
Heroin
Homeopathy
Hypnotic drugs
Immunization
Immunosuppressive drugs
Inhalants
Injections
Insulin
Intoxication
Kaolin
Laxatives

Linctus
Linaments
Local anaesthetics
LSD
Medicines
Methylated spirits
Morphine
Narcotics
Nicotine
Ointments
Oral contraceptives
Painkillers
Penicillin
Peroxide
Pharmacy
Placebo
Premedication
Preventive medicine
Proprietary
Quinine
Sedatives
Side effects
Smelling salts
Solvent abuse
Sports medicine
Steroids
Stimulants
Streptomycin
Sublingual drug
Sulpha drugs
Suppositories
Tetracycline
Thalidomide
Tranquillizers
Vaccinations

ILLNESS & TREATMENT
Anthrax
Aphasia
Appendicitis
Arteries & diseases
Arthritis
Asbestosis
Asthma
Athlete's foot
Bends
Bilharzia
Blood poisoning
Botulism
Brain damage and
  diseases
Bronchitis
Brucellosis
Bursitis
Byssinosis
Cancer
Catarrh
Cat–scratch fever
Chickenpox
Cholera
Cirrhosis
Coeliac disease
Cold sores

Common cold
Conjunctivitis
Convalescence
Convulsions
Coronary arteries &
  thrombosis
Coughs
Cyst
Cystic fibrosis
Deafness
Diabetes
Diagnosis
Diarrhoea
Diptheria
Diverticulitis
Doctors
Dysentery
Eczema
Elephantiasis
Emphysema
Encephalitis
Enteritis
Fevers
Fibrositis
Fistula
German measles
Goitre
Glandular fever
Gout

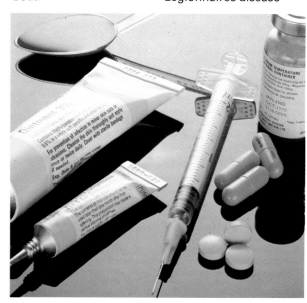

Gonorrhoea
Growths
Hay–fever
Headache
Healing
Heartburn
Heart diseases
Heat treament
Hemiplegia
Hepatitis
Hernia
Herpes
Horseness
Hodgkin's disease

Home helps
Home nursing
Home visits
Hookworm
Hospices
Hospitals
Hydatid disease
Hydrocephalus
Hydrotherapy
Hypertrophy
Hypoglycaemia
Hypothermia
Impetigo
Infarction
Infection & diseases
Inflammation
Influenza
Ingrowing toenail
Invalids
Irritable colon
Ischaemia
Kidney disease
Kwashiorkor
Kyphosis
Jaundice
Lassa fever
Legg-Calvé-Perthes
  disease
Legionnairés disease

Leprosy
Leptospirosis
Leukaemia
Leukoplakia
Light treatment
Limping
Liver diseases
Liver fluke
Loa loa
Locomotor ataxia
Lumbago
Lung disease
Lupus erythematosus,
Lymphoma

Madura foot
Malabsorption
Malaria
Malignancy
Marasmus
Marfan's syndrome
Mastoids
Measles
Ménière's disease
Meningitis
Migraine
Mitral stenosis
Motor neuron disease
Multiple sclerosis
Muscular dystrophy
Muteness
Myasthenia gravis
Mycoses
Myeloma
Myocarditis
Nausea
Nephritis
Neuralgia
Neuritis
Non–specific urethritis
Oedema
Organ removal
Osteoarthritis
Osteomyelitis
Otitis
Out–patients
Paget's disease
Paralysis
Paraplegia
Parkinson's disease
Patient's rights
Pellagra
Peptic ulcer
Pericarditis
Pernicious anaemia
Phantom limb
Phenylketonuria
Phlebitis
Phlegm
Pleurisy
Plague
Pneumoconiosis
Pneumonia
Poliomyelitis
Polycythaemia
Polyps
Proctalgia & proctitis
Prolapse
Proteinuria
Psittacosis
Psoriasis
Pulmonary disorders
Pus
Quarantine
Rabies
Radiation sickness
Raynaud's disease
Reflux
Rehabilitation
Reiter's disease
Rejection of tissue

Rheumatic fever
Rheumatism
Rheumatoid arthritis
Rhinitis
Rickets
Rickettsiae
Ringworm
St. Vitus's dance
Salmonella
Sarcoma
Scarlet fever
Sciatica
Scoliosis
Scurvy
Sensitization
Shadow
Shingles
Sickle–cell anaemia
Silicosis
Sinusitis
Skin diseases
Slipped disc
Smallpox
Sore throat
Spastics
Specimens
Speech therapy
Spondylitis
Stroke
Stye
Swelling
Synovitis
Syphilis
Tachycardia
Tennis elbow
Tetanus
Thalassaemia
Thrombosis
Thrush
Tinnitus
Total allergy syndrome
Traction
Trichnosis
Trichomoniasis
Tropical disease
Tuberculosis
Tumours
Typhoid & paratyphoid
Typhus
Ulcers
Ulcerative colitis
Uraemia
Venereal diseases
Verruca
Vitiligo
Viruses
Weil's disease
Wheezing
Whooping cough
Yellow fever

DENTAL HEALTH & HYGIENE
Abscess

Dental care
Dentist & dentistry
Dentures, crowns &
 bridges
Fluoride
Gums
Halitosis
Impacted teeth
Orthodontics
Plaque
Pyorrhoea & gingivitis
Teeth & teething

THE BODY & HOW IT WORKS
Abdomen
Adenoids
Adrenal glands
Alimentary canal
Anus
Appetite
Arteries
Autonomic nervous
 system
Balance
Bile
Birth
Bladder and bladder
 control
Blood
Blood groups
Blood pressure
Body structure
Bones
Bowel control
Brain
Breasts
Breathing
Capillaries
Cartilage
Cells & chromosomes
Circulation
Chest
Colon & colitis
Constipation
Cornea
Cramp
Diaphragm
Digestion
Dizziness
Duodenum
Dwarfism
Ears
Elbow
Endocrine system
Enzymes
Erection & ejaculation
Excretory systems
Eyes & eyesight
Face
Fatigue
Feet
Flatulence
Fontanelles

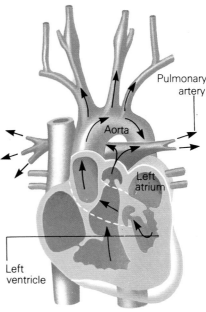

Pulmonary artery

Aorta

Left atrium

Left ventricle

Heart
Hips
Homeostasis
Hormones
Hymen
Hypothalamus
Ileum
Immune system
Intelligence
Jejunum
Joints
Keratin
Ketones
Kidney & kidney diseases
Knee
Knock knees
Gall bladder & stones
Genitals
Gigantism
Glands
Growth
Gums
Hair
Hand
Head & head injuries
Hearing
Larynx & laryngitis
Laughter
Leg
Leucocytosis
Ligaments
Lips
Lisping
Liver & liver diseases
Lordosis
Lung & lung diseases
Lymphatic system
Lymphocytes
Marrow & marrow
 transplant
Mastication
Melanin
Membranes

Memory
Menarche
Menopause
Menstruation
Metabolism
Mind
Moles
Mouth
Movement
Mucus
Muscles
Nails
Navel
Neck
Nervous system
Nose
Oesophagus
Oestrogen
Optic nerve
Orgasm
Osmosis
Ovaries
Oxygen
Pain
Palate
Pancreas
Parathyroid glands
Pelvis
Perception
Peritoneum
Perspiration
pH
Phalanges
Pharynx
Phlegm
Pins & needles
Pituitary
Placenta
Plasma
Platelets
Posture
Prostaglandins
Prostrate glands

Pulse
Rectum
Reflexes
Ribs
Saliva
Scalp
Sebaceous glands
Shin
Shivering
Shoulder
Skeleton
Skin & skin diseases
Sleep
Smell
Sneezing
Snoring
Speech
Sperm
Spinal cord
Spleen
Stomach
Subconscious
Suppuration
Taste
Teeth & teething
Temperature
Tendons
Testes
Throat
Thymus
Thyroid
Tongue
Tonsils
Tremor
Twitches
Urethra
Urine
Uterus
Uvea
Vagina
Valves
Veins
Vocal cords
Vulva
Wrists

Heredity
Identity
Imagination
Imitation
Inbreeding
Incest
Incompatibility
Infancy
Infertility
Inhibitions
Insecurity
Instinct
Intelligence
Intercourse
Introversion
Jealousy
Keeping fit
Language
Laughter
Laziness
Leisure
Libido
Listening
Loneliness
Lying
Marital problems
Mentally handicapped
    children
Middle age
Motherhood
Natural childbirth
Newborn baby
Night fears
One–parent family
Only child
Paediatrics
Parents
Play
Positive health
Post–natal depression
Precocious child
Pregnancy
Premature babies
Preventive medicine
Psychology
Questions children ask
Reading ability
Relationships
Relaxation
Separation
Sex education
Smacking
Spoilt child
Stealing
Sterilization
Substitute parents
Survival
Tantrums
Teasing
Temperament
Tenderness
Thumb–sucking
Toilet training
Truancy
Vaccinations
Weaning

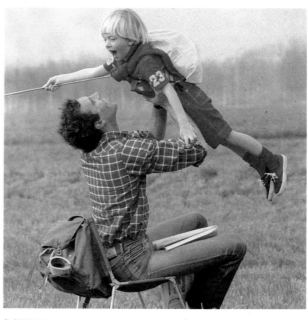

EXPLORING
PARENTHOOD
Adolescence
Attachment in infancy
Baby battering
Birth
Child development
Congenital disorders
Disturbed children
Environment
Eugenics
Family
Fantasy in childhood
Fatherhood
Feeding problems
Genetics
Growing pains
Health education

MENTAL HEALTH
Anorexia nervosa
Anxiety
Autism
Behaviour therapy
Biofeedback
Body language
Complexes &
    compulsions
Dementia
Depression
Disturbed children
Dreaming
Environment
Grief
Group therapy
Habits
Hallucinations
Head banging
Heredity
Homesickness
Hyperactivity
Hypnosis
Hypnotic drugs
Hypochondria
Hysteria
Identity
Imagination
Immaturity
Impotence
Inadequacy
Inhibitions
Insanity
Insecurity
Insomnia
Instinct
Intelligence
Introversion
Isolation
Jealousy
Kleptomania
Laziness

Lethargy
Lying
Malaise
Malingering
Mania
Manic depression
Meditation
Megalomania
Mental illness
Mentally handicapped
    children
Mind
Moods
Multiple personality
Nervous breakdown
Neurasthenia
Neuroses
Obsessions
Occupational therapy
Oedipus complex
Overcrowding
Paranoia
Perception
Personality
Phobias
Post-natal depression
Psychiatry
Psychology
Psychosomatic problems
Relationships
Relaxation
Retardation
Schizophrenia
Shyness
Stress
Subconscious
Suicide
Telepathy
Temperament
Tenderness
Tension
Withdrawal symptoms

Preface

For most doctors, establishing a strong relationship with their patients is one of the greatest rewards of practising medicine. Regrettably most of us are unable to spend as much time as we would like with each patient — explaining exactly what is happening to their bodies or providing a detailed account of the precise effect a given treatment is going to have.

This is why I welcome the publication of *The Illustrated Encyclopedia of Family Health: Doctors Answers,* a reliable guide you can turn to for advice and reassurance any time you have a question about your health. It is especially helpful to consult before you visit your doctor's surgery, so that you can use the time wisely by asking the most informed questions, and then afterwards in case you have any questions you forgot to ask, want to clear up any point you didn't understand, or need a reminder of what your doctor told you.

However, this encyclopedia is not intended to be a 'do-it-yourself' medical kit, and it most certainly cannot replace your own doctor. While every care has been taken to ensure that the information presented here is in accord with current medical knowledge, personal circumstances vary so enormously that it is not possible to be sure that all the advice given is right for every individual. Consequently, if you have any particular worry about your health, it is important to consult your doctor about it, as well as making use of the guidance *The Illustrated Encyclopedia of Family Health: Doctors Answers* can give you.

Trevor Weston, MD, MRCGP
Chief Editoral Consultant

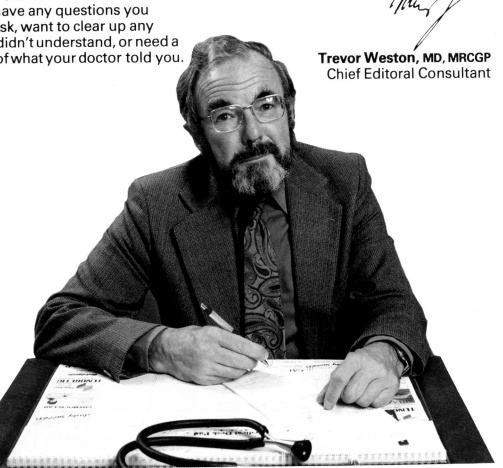

Kleptomania
Knee
Knock knees
Kwashiorkor
Kyphosis
Lacerations

Laminectomy
Language
Laparoscopy
Laparotomy
Larynx and laryngitis
Lasers

Lassa fever
Laughter
Laxatives
Laziness
Lazy eye
Lead poisoning

Learning
Leg
Legg-Calvé-Perthes
   disease
Legionnaire's disease
Leisure

Volume 10

Leprosy
Leptospirosis
Lesbianism
Lethargy
Leucocytosis
Leucorrhoea
Leucotomy
Leukaemia
Leukoplakia
Libido
Lice
Lichen

Life expectancy
Lifting
Ligaments
Lighting
Lightning accidents
Light treatments
Limping
Linctus
Liniments
Lipoma
Lips
Liquid diet
Lisping
Listening

Lithotomy
Liver and liver diseases
Liver fluke
Liver spots
Loa loa
Local anaesthetics
Lochia
Locomotor ataxia
Loneliness
Longevity
Lordosis
LSD
Lumbago
Lumbar puncture

Lung and lung disease
Lupus erythematosus
Lying
Lymphatic system
Lymphocytes
Lymphoma
Macrobiotics
Madura foot
Magnesium
Malabsorption
Malaise
Malaria

Volume 11

Male menopause
Malignancy
Malingering
Mallet finger
Malnutrition
Malt
Mania
Manic depression
Manipulation
Mantoux test

Marasmus
Marfan's syndrome
Marital problems
Marrow and transplants
Massage
Mastectomy
Mastication
Mastitis
Mastoids
Masturbation
Measles
Meconium

Medical ethics
Medical research
Medical technology
Medicines
Meditation
Megacolon
Megalomania
Melanin
Membranes
Memory
Menarche
Ménière's disease

Meningitis
Menopause
Menstruation
Mental illness
Mentally handicapped
   children
Metabolism
Methylated spirit
Microbiology
Microsurgery
Middle age

Volume 12

Midwifery
Migraine
Milk
Mind
Minerals
Miscarriage
Mites
Mitral stenosis
Moles

Mongolism
Monitoring equipment
Monosodium glutamate
Moods
Morning sickness
Morphine
Motherhood
Motor neuron disease
Mountain sickness
Mouth
Movement

Mucus
Multiple birth
Multiple personality
Multiple sclerosis
Mumps
Murmurs of the heart
Muscles
Muscular dystrophy
Mushroom poisoning
Mutation
Muteness

Myasthenia gravis
Mycoses
Myeloma
Myocarditis
Nails
Nappy rash
Narcotics
Natural childbirth
Naturopathy
Nausea

Volume 13

Navel
Neck
Nephrectomy
Nephritis
Nervous breakdown
Nervous system
Nettle sting
Neuralgia
Neurasthenia

Neuritis
Neurology and
   neurosurgery
Neuroses
Newborn baby
Nicotine
Night blindness
Night fears
Nits
Noise
Non-specific urethritis

Nose
Numbness
Nursery
Nursing
Nursing homes
Nutrition
Nystagmus
Obesity
Obsessions
Obstetrics
Obstructions

Occupational hazards
Occupational therapy
Oedema
Oedipus complex
Oesophagus
Oestrogen
Ointments
Old age
One-parent families

Volume 14

Only child
Open-heart surgery

Operating theatre
Ophthalmology

Optician
Optic nerve

Contents

A-vitamin

Q What are vitamins? Are they really important?

A Vitamins are organic substances present in minute amounts in food. Put simply, they help make our bodies work. Because they cannot be made by the body, vitamins must be obtained from the diet. We require only very small amounts of them, but they are absolutely essential to normal metabolism, and a serious deficiency will inevitably lead to disease.

Q Should I take vitamin supplements to make sure I don't develop a vitamin deficiency?

A Children, the elderly, pregnant women and nursing mothers, as well as people recovering from an illness, may need a supplement of certain vitamins. A healthy adult, though, will usually obtain enough through a well-balanced diet.

Q I know a daily dose of halibut liver oil is good for children. Is a double dose twice as good?

A Halibut liver oil is a valuable source of vitamin A, but it is dangerous to exceed the recommended dose. Because vitamin A is stored in the body, excessive amounts can be toxic.

Q I've heard that vitamin A helps prevent colds. Is there any truth to this?

A Vitamin A aids the body in producing mucus-secreting cells, and this is one of the ways the body protects itself from germs. It works by removing them from the body—by the nose in the case of a cold. So a lack of vitamin A could make you more likely to catch colds.

Q Will eating carrots help me see in the dark, or is this just an old wives' tale?

A There is some truth in this old wives' tale. The carotene contained in carrots provides vitamin A, which helps your eyes to adjust to dim light quickly.

We have all heard of vitamins and know they are essential for good health. But what are they, what do they do and, among them, just how important is vitamin A?

Vitamin A is one of the vital group of vitamins that the body needs to function properly. It enables us to see in a dim light, keeps our skin healthy, ensures normal growth and renews the body tissue. With only a few exceptions, we obtain all the vitamins we need from our food, and the minute amounts the body requires mostly exist in their natural state in food. But vitamin A is largely manufactured by the body from a food substance called carotene.

Sources of vitamin A
The vitamin A in our food comes in two different forms from two different sources. The pure form, called retinol, is found in foods such as fish-liver oils, liver, kidney, cheese, eggs and butter, having already been manufactured by the animal concerned. The second form we make ourselves from carotene, which is found in such vegetables as carrots, spinach, cabbage, and tomatoes.

In fact, when a vegetable is orange, yellow or dark green in colour, what you are seeing is its carotene content, and the darker the green of the vegetable, the greater the carotene content. Spinach and watercress therefore contain more in each pound than cabbage, and dark green cabbage provides more than lighter types of vegetable.

Carotene is converted into retinol in the liver and in the small intestine, and then some of the vitamin A—whether it be converted carotene or retinol itself—is absorbed into the blood stream and circulated round the body to be used in its everyday functions, while the rest is stored in the liver.

Although vitamin A is not present in many foods, those which contain it are fortunately readily available. A fifth of our average intake comes from vegetables, mainly carrots. Turnips and potatoes are no substitute, however, since they contain no carotene. Milk and butter are other common sources; margarine, to which vitamin A is added artificially, contains almost as much as butter and is therefore just as good.

Vitamin A-rich foods tend not to lose their vitamin content easily, though prolonged exposure to light and air can reduce the amount. Cooking at normal temperatures has no serious effect, but frying at a relatively high temperature in butter or margarine will result in some loss of vitamin content.

Vitamin A deficiency
Itching, burning and reddened eyelids are among the problems caused by lack of vitamin A, and a drastic deficiency can lead to blindness. The children of the poorer nations are most vulnerable and the cause is early weaning on to an unsuitable food like skimmed milk, which contains no vitamins at all. However, prepared baby foods almost always have essential vitamins added to them.

In our more affluent society our diet is better balanced, and most of us get as much vitamin A as we need, about two-thirds of it coming from retinol and one-third from carotene.

But even so, a deficiency of vitamin A can cause night blindness. Doctors have long recognized night blindness as a medical condition. Normally, it takes about seven to ten minutes for your eyes to become used to a dim light—so if you are dazzled for some time after seeing another car's headlights at night, or if you find it difficult to distinguish objects in the semi-dark, see your doctor to find out if you have vitamin A deficiency. Taking halibut liver oil capsules is the quickest cure, as it is one of the best sources of vitamin A.

If you are on a high protein diet you could risk a deficiency simply because the body uses up the vitamin much faster when converting protein into body tissue and energy. But there are other times when the body uses up its store of vitamin A too quickly, such as when there is a high fever.

Taking certain drugs also causes a loss. Your doctor will advise you as to how much vitamin A is needed should any of these situations arise.

Excessive vitamin A
The forty or so vitamins can be divided into two types—those that can be stored by the body and those that cannot. As vitamin A is stored in the liver daily intake is not essential though regular supplies are needed. There is some danger however in taking too much vitamin A. This is very unlikely to result from intake through food but can occur if large amounts are taken in concentrated forms such as halibut liver oil capsules. Symptoms may include insomnia, weight loss, dryness of the lips, and aching limbs. But, in general, taking slightly more than is needed is unlikely to harm you or your child.

Vitamin A—Are you getting enough?

The daily requirement for different age groups and the vitamin A content in the foods listed are given in micrograms (1,000 micrograms = one milligram, or one thousandth of a gram).

There is no need to worry if you are unable to take the correct amount every day as long as the amount you take over a week gives the correct daily average.

Age group		Daily requirement
Babies under 12 months		450
Children	1-6	300
	7-8	400
	9-11	575·
Adolescents		750
Adult men and women		750
Expectant mothers		
first 4 months		750
until the birth		900
during breastfeeding		1,200

Food	Vitamin A content
Apricots, dried, 57 g (2 oz)	340
Butter, 28 g (1 oz)	282
Cabbage, 114 g (4 oz)	56
Carrots, 114 g (4 oz)	2267
Cheese, 57 g (2 oz)	238
Cod liver oil capsule, 1	180
Cream, heavy, 2 tablespoons (30 ml)	130
Egg, 1	80
Halibut liver oil capsule, 1	1200

Food	Vitamin A content
Kidney, 114 g (4 oz)	340
Fish, oily, 114 g (4 oz)	52
Liver, ox, 114 g (4 oz)	6800
Margarine, 28 g (1 oz)	255
Milk, whole, .2 L (7 fl oz)	80
Peas, frozen, 114 g (4 oz)	56
Prunes, dried, 57 g (2 oz)	90
Spinach, 114 g (4 oz)	1136
Tomato, 42 g (1½ oz)	49
Watercress, 28 g (1 oz)	142

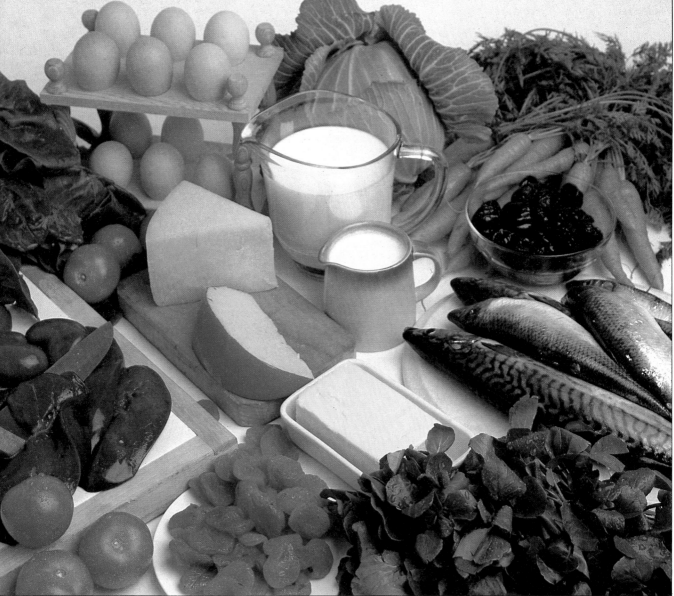

Di Lewis

Abdomen

Q I went for a job interview the other day and my tummy rumbled all the time. I was so embarrassed. As I didn't get the job, how can I avoid the problem next time?

A Tummy rumblings go on all the time as the intestine churns and digests food, but cannot usually be heard except through a stethoscope. Louder rumblings tend to occur when the intestine is empty or contains too much air. You were probably a little bit nervous at the prospect of your interview, and when people are nervous they often swallow air without realizing it. So next time, have a good meal before you set off, try to relax and suck a peppermint or two to help prevent you from air swallowing.

Q My child often complains of a tummy ache on Monday mornings. It seems odd that it's only then. Is she just shamming?

A Quite probably she does have a real pain in her abdomen caused not by some sort of infection but by nerves. The pain, though real, is probably caused by a mental rather than a physical problem. Try to find out why Mondays are so much to be dreaded. Perhaps she is being bullied or is afraid of one of her teachers. Once you get to the root of the problems and iron out her anxieties, the trouble should disappear very quickly.

Q My baby seems to have a huge abdomen, just like one of those starving children I've seen on television. Is this normal?

A Quite normal. A baby's abdomen looks swollen because his liver is very large—it has to be to do many of the important jobs essential to growth, for example making blood—and the abdominal muscles are not yet very strong. By the time he is about five he should have lost this 'pot bellied' look. Starving children have swollen abdomens whatever their age. This is a part of a disease called kwashiorkor caused by a diet containing little or no protein. Such children do not have sturdy limbs like your baby but arms and legs so wasted that they look like matchsticks.

The abdomen is the factory area of the body, containing most of the digestive system, the urinary system and, in women, the reproductive organs. With all these activities going on inside, it is not surprising that pains in the abdomen can have a huge variety of causes.

The abdomen is the biggest cavity in the body, extending from underneath the diaphragm, the sheet of muscle that forms the lower boundary of the chest, down to the groin. Bounded at the back of the body by the spine, and round its upper sides by the ribs, the front of the abdomen is covered by a thick sheet of muscle which can be felt just by 'pulling it in'. And it is easy to realize just how elastic this muscle is by picturing how much it can stretch to accommodate a baby during pregnancy.

Inside the abdomen
There are a great number of organs in the abdomen, often called the viscera. Nearly all the alimentary canal lies inside the abdomen, starting with the stomach sited just under the diaphragm and ending with the rectum, which empties out via the anus. The alimentary canal is the body's food processing system—it breaks down food into substances that can be absorbed into the blood to be carried to all parts of the body, and ejects indigestible wastes. Backing up the alimentary canal

Female abdomen with alimentary canal removed

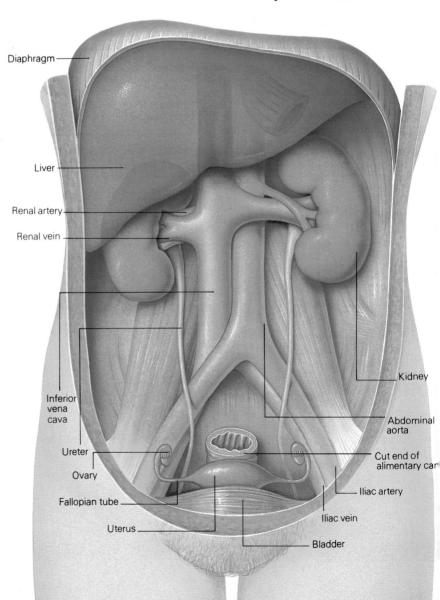

Diaphragm

Liver

Renal artery

Renal vein

Kidney

Inferior vena cava

Abdominal aorta

Ureter

Cut end of alimentary can

Ovary

Iliac artery

Fallopian tube

Iliac vein

Uterus

Bladder

Mike Courteney

4

are important abdominal glands such as the liver and pancreas, plus the spleen, which is part of the defence system against disease. A huge network of blood vessels serves all the abdominal organs and nerves.

Behind the alimentary canal lie the kidneys, each joined by a tube called a ureter to the bladder, which is in the lower part of the abdomen and in which urine is stored before it is released. Closely connected to the urinary system is the reproductive system. In women, nearly all the sex organs are inside the abdomen, but in men part of the sex organs descend to a position outside the body before birth.

It might seem impossible for so many vital organs to be squeezed into such a comparatively small space, but through the centuries of evolution the 10 m (33 ft) or so of gut have become coiled and twisted to fit inside the abdomen. To keep everything in place, the abdomen is lined with a kind of tissue sac called the peritoneum and the organs are attached to it by sheets or strings of tissue known as mesenteries.

When something goes wrong
With so much going on inside the

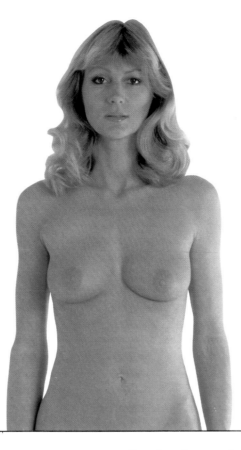

abdomen, it is perhaps just as well that, apart from the odd rumble of the intestines, it is impossible to feel each organ at work. But because we cannot feel them working, we cannot actually detect when anything goes wrong, except 'by proxy' in some other part of the body. Thus the pain of a stomach ulcer, for example, is real enough but it is not in the stomach itself that the pain is felt but in nerve signals reaching the upper part of the abdomen.

Pains in the abdomen vary in position, type and intensity according to the cause of the trouble within and are in themselves good clues for the doctor's diagnosis. The pains are usually accompanied by other symptoms—nausea, vomiting and/or diarrhoea, as for instance in the case of food poisoning. And diseases of the abdominal organs can also be detected by pains in other parts of the body such as the back and shoulders.

Sex-linked symptoms
Many women become concerned about an uncomfortable, low abdominal pain which they get midway between periods. This is in fact perfectly normal, and it isn't worth bothering the doctor with unless the pain persists for more than 24 hours or is accompanied by bleeding.

Common causes of abdominal pain

Position	Type of pain/symptoms	Possible causes	What to do
Top centre, behind breastbone	Severe discomfort, or burning sensation. Nausea and headache. Heavy feeling in abdomen which may be distended. Wind or heartburn.	Inflammation of stomach due to infection, excess of rich or spicy food, alcohol or nicotine. Peptic ulcer or chronic gastritis	Take antacids, plenty of fluids, eat a bland diet. Cut down on drinking and smoking, try to avoid stress. See your doctor if pain persists
Top centre, moving through to back	Colicky (griping), persistent or intermittent, may be relieved by food. Upper part of abdomen may feel full and be distended	Peptic ulcer or inflammation of the pancreas	Take antacids for temporary relief, plus small milky meals, but see your doctor this week
Top centre, behind ribs, moving to right	Constant, may be made worse by fatty foods. Heartburn, abdomen feels oppressively full. Possibly jaundiced	Inflamed gall bladder, inflammation of liver (hepatitis)	See your doctor today
Top centre, shooting to right shoulder	Agonizing, with sweating, nausea and vomiting	Trapped gall stones (biliary colic)	See your doctor urgently, take painkillers for temporary relief
Centre, around or above navel	Persistent, may be burning, cramping or griping, often accompanied by vomiting and/or diarrhoea. Abdomen distended	Food poisoning, gastro-enteritis or other infection of the intestine	Take plenty of fluid and kaolin and morphine mixture. No food for 24 hours. See your doctor if symptoms persist
Centre or in either loin, may shoot down to groin; burning on urination	Colicky or persistent, may be worse on movement and accompanied by vomiting	Kidney infection or stone (renal colic)	See your doctor today, or at once if pain is very severe
Centre, round navel, moving to lower right	Persistent, may be accompanied by flatulence, nausea and vomiting. Constipation	Appendicitis	See your doctor today, or at once if pain is very severe. Do not take laxatives or antacids

The pain is actually caused by an increase in tension in the ovary as the egg is released halfway between each menstrual period. Many women do not have this pain at all but wish that they did—for it is quite an accurate indication of when the egg is being released and therefore when a woman is most likely to get pregnant.

Also connected with reproduction, but rather more unusual, is the set of symptoms known as couvade. Occasionally it is possible for a man whose wife is pregnant to suffer some of the same symptoms as a pregnant woman. The condition is caused by extreme over-anxiety, and the man suffers abdominal swelling and also sometimes morning sickness and food cravings. After the birth the abdomen invariably returns to normal.

When to seek help

Abdominal pains are something that everyone has experienced, but it is important to remember that although they often have a trivial cause, such as over-eating, constipation or a mild 'tummy bug', they can be a signal that something is seriously wrong. Abdominal pain should always be taken seriously and should not just be masked with pain killers, which can actually cover up important symptoms that require a

Intestinal organs

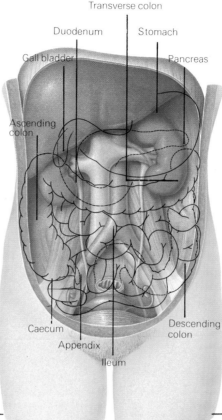

Transverse colon
Duodenum
Stomach
Gall bladder
Pancreas
Ascending colon
Caecum
Descending colon
Appendix
Ileum

doctor's immediate attention and care.

In obvious, everyday complaints, wait 48 hours before seeking medical help, but in severe, sudden abdominal pain never just 'grin and bear it' or take pain-killers or laxatives. If an intense pain lasts more than a few hours, and particularly if it is accompanied by a swollen abdomen that feels tender to the touch and by blood or tarry substances in the motions, *see a doctor at once*. This is most important—don't feel you are wasting his time. It could be the sign of serious illness.

Treating children's pains

All the same rules apply if children have pains in the abdomen, but if in doubt, always consult your doctor. In children abdominal pain may also result from problems uncommon in adult life. Good examples are tonsillitis, middle ear infections and lead poisoning from chewing lead-containing paint.

Anxiety is another common cause of tummy ache in both children and adults—and results from the natural tendency of the body to intensify the squeezing action of the intestine in times of stress. If possible it is best not to eat at times like these because food is particularly hard to digest when the abdomen is tight. But hot drinks may bring some comfort and relief.

Position	Type of pain/symptoms	Possible causes	What to do
Centre, above, around or just below navel, right or left	Griping. Abdomen may be distended. Hard motions may alternate with diarrhoea	Constipation, irritable colon, or diverticulitis	Increase bran and roughage content of diet. See your doctor if symptoms persist
Centre, around and below navel	Cramping with frequent vomiting and constipation. Abdomen distended	Intestinal obstruction	See your doctor urgently
Centre, below navel	Griping, intermittent. Abdomen may be distended	Inflammation of the colon, miscarriage or passing of a blood clot from the vagina	See your doctor today
Centre, below navel	Persistent, occurring during or just before menstruation. Abdomen may be distended	Premenstrual tension, period pain	Take pain killers but see your doctor if symptoms persist or become severe
Below navel, right or left	Persistent dull ache, worse during periods, lower abdomen may be distended	Congestion in area of the uterus, inflammation of pelvic or sex organs, venereal disease	See your doctor this week
Below navel, right or left	Colicky, intermittent, accompanying scanty or missed periods	Ectopic pregnancy (foetus lodged in the Fallopian tubes)	See your doctor today
Very low, centre, may move down into groin	Constant, may be worse as bladder fills. Burning sensation during urination, urine may be thick or contain blood	Cystitis or urinary infection	See your doctor today. Take plenty of fluids
All over abdomen	Agonizing, rapid onset, very tender all over abdomen. Generally very ill, possibly collapsed	Peritonitis from perforated peptic ulcer or burst appendix	Call a doctor or get to hospital urgently

Abortion

Q Is it dangerous to have a number of abortions? I have heard that it is.

A Yes, it can be, because there is a real risk of sterility from having *repeated* abortions. The cervix (neck of the womb) can become stretched, making it easier for germs to enter the womb. As a result, the Fallopian tubes may become blocked due to infection, so the eggs released by the ovaries cannot reach the womb to be fertilized. Stretching of the cervix can also lead to miscarriage, though a stitch across the opening of the cervix can usually—but not always—retain the foetus to its full term.

Q I had an abortion as a teenager. Now I am about to have a medical which involves an internal examination. Will the doctor be able to tell that I have had an abortion?

A This is not very likely—especially if it was an early abortion carried out by vacuum suction. In any case, there is no need to worry even if he does find evidence. A doctor is bound to keep all medical information about you confidential.

Q What should I do if I have excessive bleeding after an abortion?

A See your doctor immediately.

Q I have heard that having an abortion can make you infertile. Is there any truth in this?

A No, only if the operation goes wrong, and that rarely happens these days. In fact, current medical thinking suggests that, in some cases, the woman can be *more* fertile afterwards. This is because the lining of the womb may be scraped away during the D and C type of abortion, and a fertilized egg is more likely to attach itself to a new lining than an old one. A woman having trouble conceiving is sometimes advised to have a 'scrape'. With the vacuum method of abortion, however, a woman is only as likely to become pregnant as she would be normally, since it is the contents of the womb that are removed, not the lining.

Nobody likes the idea of abortion. But the woman who thinks she needs one should understand what is involved and how to get sympathetic counselling and help.

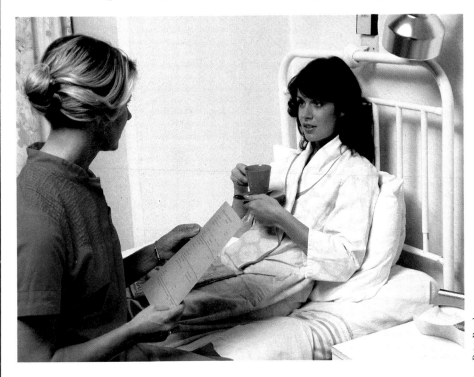

Peter Dazely

Doctors refer to any ending of pregnancy before the 28th week, even if it is due to natural causes, as abortion, but to most people abortion means the artificial termination of an unwanted pregnancy. Once, abortion meant a sordid and risky backstreet procedure, but today women who need a termination can usually have one safely in a hospital or clinic.

However, there are laws against indiscriminate abortions and abortion should never be regarded as a substitute for contraception. Generally, each case has to be judged on its merits and two independent medical opinions are usually required before an abortion can be performed.

Reasons for an abortion
These can be roughly divided into the social and the medical. The most common non-medical reason is that the pregnancy was unplanned and unwanted. It may have resulted from contraceptive failure (or no contraception at all), from a casual affair, or even from rape. Other reasons include unfavourable circumstances, such as inadequate housing, a low income, or an unstable relationship between the couple.

In some cases, the pregnant woman may already have all the children she can cope with, or she may be in her forties and view a late baby with alarm. On the other

Today's legal abortions, performed early, are practically risk-free and the after-effects are minimal.

hand, a pregnant teenager may not be willing or able to bring up a child.

The main medical reasons for abortion concern the risk of mental or physical abnormality in the baby or the possibility of harm to the mother if the pregnancy continues. Abortion is generally recommended if German measles (rubella) has been contracted in the first three months.

Abortion may also be suggested where spina bifida (a serious defect of the spinal cord) or chromosome disorders, such as Down's syndrome (which causes a child to be born mentally defective), are detected.

Counselling
Any woman who feels she should have an abortion will need to discuss the matter with someone. Counselling before any decision on a termination is taken is essential. Many women have very confused feelings about abortion and require professional guidance.

Sometimes the solution may be to have the baby adopted. This decision can be the right one for a woman who may feel that abortion is morally wrong. And sometimes the troubles and fears that a woman gives as her reasons for wanting

7

Q Why is abortion recommended if a woman has contracted German measles during early pregnancy?

A If it has been contracted in the first three months of pregnancy there is a definite risk that the virus will have attacked the developing foetus and that the baby will be born blind or deaf or be mentally affected.

Q I have been thinking about having an abortion and feel I must discuss it with someone—but who?

A It is very important to talk it over with your partner—he may be able to put your feelings in perspective. Also your family, friends and relatives can sometimes be surprisingly sympathetic and helpful, though because of a lack of professional knowledge, their advice may be misleading and in the end not what's right for you. Your best bet is to contact someone who is trained to help in situations like these: your doctor, a gynaecologist, social worker, psychiatrist, priest, or one of the advisors at a family planning clinic or pregnancy bureau. They will be able to explain exactly what an abortion involves and can help you get one, if that is what you really want.

Q I am ten weeks pregnant and about to have an abortion. How long must I stay in hospital?

A Performed any time within the first three months, an abortion usually only involves an overnight stay in a clinic or hospital and, in some areas, out-patient abortions are available where the woman is at the clinic or in hospital for only a few hours.

Q When can I expect to be fully recovered after an abortion?

A Menstruation can return to normal the following month, but in most cases it takes a month or two to resume a regular pattern. Intercourse should be postponed for at least two weeks—longer if possible. And it is possible to become pregnant again very soon, so contraception is necessary.

an abortion can be alleviated by counselling. However, a woman who really wants and needs an abortion will always receive help.

How abortions are carried out

Early abortions, when the pregnancy is in its initial stages of development, are quicker, easier and much preferred by patients, doctors and nursing staff. After four to five months the foetus begins to move, and abortions at this stage may be followed by lactation (milk flow) which can be extremely distressing.

Two methods are currently used to carry out an early abortion. The first, D and E (dilation and evacuation), which is more commonly known as either vacuum suction or vacuum curettage, is carried out when the foetus is between seven and 12 weeks old.

The second abortion technique is a D and C (dilation and curettage). This is generally used for pregnancies of between eight and 12 weeks, but this can be extended to 15 weeks in some cases.

After the first three months of preg-

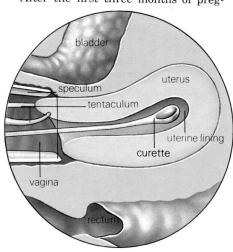

Dilation and curettage method

Early abortions can be carried out by D&E (right), which takes ten minutes under general anaesthetic. The vagina is opened with a speculum and the exact depth of the womb (uterus) measured. The neck of the womb (cervix) is then gently opened. A tentaculum holds it open and the tip of a vacurette (a rigid tube) is inserted. This is attached to a suction pump which frees and draws out the foetal material along with the early afterbirth. D&C (above) is done in the same way except that a curette (a metal loop with a handle) loosens the foetal material, which is removed from the uterus with forceps. The scale diagram (far right) shows the size of the female reproductive organs in relation to the whole body.

nancy, other methods have to be used. But whereas in the early stages the methods used are relatively safe, late abortion does have an element of risk.

Such late abortions (sometimes called a prostaglandin abortion) are carried out at about 16 to 28 weeks. Because the foetus is no longer small enough to be extracted by suction or curettage, an abortion-inducing solution is injected, usually vaginally but sometimes via a drip, into the amniotic sac, known as the 'bag-of-waters', surrounding the foetus. This causes the patient to go into labour so that the abortion occurs through the natural process of delivery.

Before 16 weeks, the sac is not large enough to be located accurately, so this process of inducing labour by injections into the amniotic sac cannot be used safely before this time. A more recent method introduces a solution—usually in the form of prostaglandin pessaries—into the top of the vagina close to the womb, rather than the sac. This has proved effective in bringing on labour and has few side-effects.

There is a last method of carrying out a late abortion (16 to 28 weeks). Called a hysterotomy (not to be confused with hysterectomy), it is only used when induction methods have proved unsuccessful. As in a caesarean section, the foetus is removed through a small incision in the abdomen, usually just below the pubic

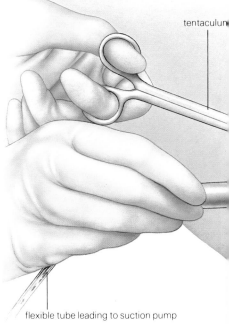

flexible tube leading to suction pump

Dilation and evacuation metho

hairline. However, this technique has the highest risk of complications and it can sometimes limit a woman to caesarean births in the future. It also involves several days' stay in hospital.

After-effects

There is very little danger attached to having an abortion in a hospital or clinic. The real danger is to the woman who goes to the back-street abortionist—where she could run the risk of infection, a punctured womb and even death.

But there are a few minor side-effects which can occur after even the most well-conducted abortion. A woman who is too energetic during the 48 hours following the operation may find she experiences heavy bleeding, and this will require bedrest. Blood loss following abortion varies from woman to woman: it may finish after a few days, like a period, or it may go on for two or three weeks. Some women get intermittent cramp pains for a few days afterwards.

Sudden pain, excessive bleeding, or a rise in temperature after abortion should always be reported to your doctor. But these symptoms only rarely occur and they can be treated so long as your doctor is consulted immediately.

Because the cervix will remain open for a while after most types of abortion, there is a slight risk of infection. If an infection spreads to the Fallopian tubes it could result in infertility. To reduce this risk, tampons or any other internal protection must not be used to staunch bleeding until after the first period has passed. Instead use sterile sanitary towels.

Some doctors also recommend not sitting or lying in a bath after the operation, though kneeling upright is all right.

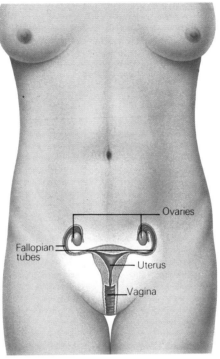

Mike Courteney

Reassurance

After all abortions, final counselling should include contraceptive advice to avoid further need for terminations. In the case of the older woman who has completed her family, counselling should include discussion of sterilization for her or a vasectomy for her husband.

Occasionally, psychological effects are felt after abortion and these may be more likely after late abortion. Such emotional upsets may involve a sense of guilt and can lead to depression and a sense of loss or bereavement. This is not abnormal, and no woman should feel that, because abortions are relatively simple, she should just be able to breeze through it without any emotion. A great deal will depend on the circumstances that dictated the abortion, on the attitude of the partner, family and friends, and on the quality of the counselling before the decision was taken. Emotional support is a vital part of the care a woman who is having an abortion needs.

If you are pregnant and think you need an abortion

DO

● see your doctor as soon as your period is two weeks overdue. There can be many reasons for a missed period, and only a pregnancy test or an internal examination can tell you if you're expecting a baby.

● take a positive attitude. Abortion is not a shameful matter today and the people who are there to help you will not try to make you feel guilty.

● consider alternatives, such as adoption, before making a decision. Your doctor or a professional counsellor can give guidance.

DON'T

● try old-fashioned 'remedies'—throwing yourself down stairs, for example, or gin and hot baths. You could injure yourself severely—and still be pregnant.

● under any circumstances go to a back-street abortionist. You could suffer irreparable damage and still be pregnant.

● listen to myths, such as 'If you have an abortion, you'll never feel much pleasure in love-making again', or, 'You'll always have difficult pregnancies once you've had an abortion'. They are nonsense.

Female reproductive organs

Frank Kennard

Abrasions and cuts

Q Is it better to cover wounds or let them heal in the open air?

A As a general rule, all wet, weepy wounds need covering. Most fresh wounds are best protected if you are working in dirty conditions, but dry wounds should be left uncovered in clean conditions.

Q Do old people heal as quickly as the young?

A Generally, older bodies heal just as quickly as young ones, but there are a few exceptions. Sometimes arterial disease diminishes the blood flow and makes healing a slow process. Infection is more likely and ulcers may develop, especially on the shins and ankles, where circulation is often bad. Cuts on an elderly person's leg need prompt, daily attention if ulcers are to be avoided.

Q If a limb is bleeding severely, should I try to make a tourniquet?

A Tourniquets—strips of cloth or other material wrapped tightly around a limb—stop bleeding by cutting off the blood supply. They were once widely used but are now thought to be dangerous because a low blood and oxygen level in any limb can cause permanent damage and make infection more likely. Tourniquets should only be used by a qualified person.

Q Do I need a tetanus injection every time I get cut?

A Like most people you will probably have been immunized against tetanus as a child. Immunization involves having a series of three injections within a year. To maintain protection you should have a booster every ten years. If you have not had one in the last ten years (five years if the wound is very serious) you will need to have a small booster injection if you are cut. An injection is particularly important if you were cut while gardening or in the countryside, as the bacteria which cause tetanus live in soil and animal manure. If you are uncertain whether you have been immunized seek medical advice. Tetanus germs cause lockjaw, a very serious condition that is often fatal.

The skin protects vulnerable internal organs from injury, but as the body's front line of defence it often gets damaged itself. Fast, effective first aid can help speed the healing process and prevent infection.

Scratches, abrasions, cuts, lacerations and punctures are all abnormal breaks through the skin and are generally referred to as wounds. The body itself has very efficient mechanisms for staunching bleeding, healing wounds and fighting infection, but it often needs help. Whenever the skin is broken blood vessels may be torn and germs can enter the body, so all wounds need to be cleaned and many need to be dressed.

How the body copes

Blood contains special proteins that form a protective mesh of strands and cells when tissue is damaged. Called a blood clot, it seals off the broken blood vessels and stops bleeding. At the same time the muscles in the walls of the damaged blood vessels contract to slow down the flow of blood. If bleeding is severe the blood pressure is lowered throughout the body.

Also, as soon as skin is broken, special white blood cells called phagocytes gather at the site of injury. They remove any microscopic particles like bacteria and so are the body's first line of defence against infection. As expected, the larger the damaged area the more likely it will be contaminated with bacteria and the greater the chance of infection.

When bleeding has stopped and the wound is clear of infection, a fibrous scab begins to form. The scab shrinks over the next few days and forms an extremely strong bond between the cut surfaces.

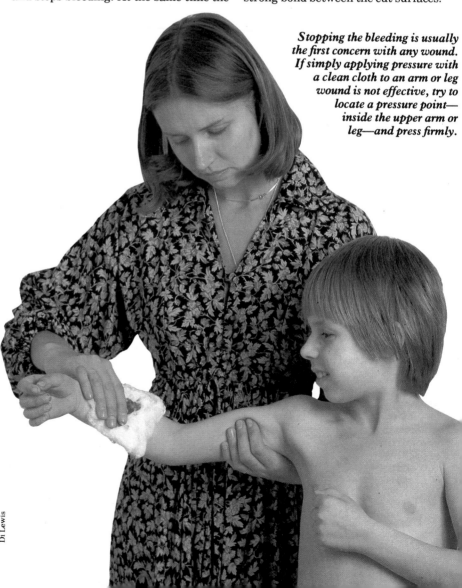

Stopping the bleeding is usually the first concern with any wound. If simply applying pressure with a clean cloth to an arm or leg wound is not effective, try to locate a pressure point— inside the upper arm or leg—and press firmly.

Di Lewis

First aid for minor injuries

FIRST AID

How to stop bleeding

Sometimes it is better to allow a wound to bleed for a while because the flow of blood can help to wash dirt and bacteria away. This is particularly important with a puncture wound, as these are very difficult to clean properly. However if bleeding is profuse, it should be stopped.

Unless you suspect a broken limb, in which case the limb should not be moved, raise the limb so that the blood pressure is reduced slightly.

Then, using a clean bandage, apply firm pressure to the wound. The pressure needs to be constant for at least five minutes to be effective. If blood seeps through the bandage, don't change it, just add more on top: dabbing a wound or changing a bandage removes any blood clot.

If blood is flowing with a pumping, squirting movement, an artery has been damaged. In this case medical help should be sought immediately,

but in the meantime continue to apply firm pressure. If you locate the local artery and press on it, this will be effective, but not for longer than 15 minutes at a time.

One exception: although scalp wounds bleed profusely, do not apply direct pressure if you suspect a skull fracture. Instead build up a dressing in the shape of a ring so that the pressure is applied around the wound, but not directly on it.

Cleaning wounds

Before you prepare to clean the wound, cover it with a clean cloth so that no more germs can enter it. Then wash your hands thoroughly, taking special care to scrub under the nails.

Wounds can be cleaned with a variety of liquids, from mild antiseptics to soap and water or mild detergents and water. Tap water is quite sterile, so it is not essential to boil water in a kettle.

If you use any antiseptic other than hydrogen peroxide BP, which is safe to use straight from the bottle, be sure to dilute it as instructed on the bottle. Using too strong a solution may damage the tissues and make the wound worse.

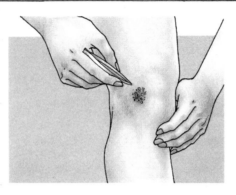

If there is any grit in the wound, a quick scrub with a clean brush under running water is an effective though painful way of removing it. Large pieces of grit and splinters should be removed individually with a pair of tweezers. If a large splinter will not lift out easily, it should be left until further medical care is given.

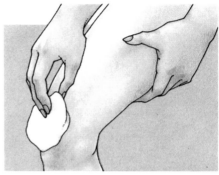

Brush any last bits of dirt from the surface of the wound with small swabs of gauze or cotton wool soaked in antiseptic. Then, working away from the wound, clean around it using fresh antiseptic swabs. Finally, clean the wound itself using separate swabs for every stroke. Work from the centre out.

Applying a dressing

A small, clean cut can be covered with 'butterfly' plasters. These are specially prepared, thin strips of adhesive plaster used to hold the wound closed. The strips should be placed diagonally across each other, pulling the edges of the wound together.

A non-stick dressing is the best protection for a small wound as it can be removed without harming the scab. Never use cotton wool or the woolly side of lint as this sticks to the wound. Large wounds should be covered with sterile gauze dressings that take in the skin surrounding the wound as well.

Nigel Osborne

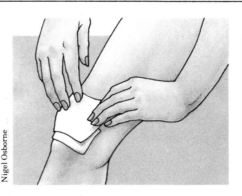

Then pad the dressing with cotton wool or additional layers of gauze: these will absorb any discharge and act as a protecting buffer. When the dressing is changed the layers should be peeled off individually.

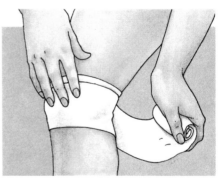

Wrap the whole area firmly with a cotton or crepe bandage. Crepe is stretchy so it fits around awkward shapes easily. Dressings should be changed regularly. If the dressing has stuck to the wound, soak it off in a mild antiseptic solution. Never pull it off quickly as this will damage the scab.

Types of wound

There are five different types of wound: scratches, abrasions, cuts, lacerations and punctures. A scratch is a superficial tear through the outer layer of the skin called the epidermis. The edges of the skin are not separated and the small amount of bleeding comes from the tiny blood vessels within the skin itself. A scratch stops bleeding quickly but it is still a site for potential infection, especially if the skin is scratched by something dirty.

Abrasions

An abrasion is an area of skin that has been torn away by force. Light scuffing of the skin is called a graze, but sometimes a large, deep area of skin is affected and the abrasion is more like a severe burn. Occasionally an abrasion is so severe that a skin graft is needed some time later. Abrasions can be much more painful than cuts as millions of tiny nerve endings are exposed. They are nearly always full of dirt or grit, so the main problem is infection. After thoroughly cleaning the abrasion to remove dirt and grit, cover it with dry gauze until a scab forms.

Cuts

Any clean division through the layers of the skin is called a cut. Cuts are usually caused by sharp edges such as glass, razors, kitchen knives or even paper. They often bleed quite freely, especially if a deep cut damages large blood vessels underneath the skin, but this can usually be controlled.

Many cuts tend to gape slightly, so to aid the healing process keep the edges together with a butterfly plaster or porous synthetic surgical tape placed across the cut. This is especially advisable for cuts on the elbows or knees, which are constantly being bent, and on the fingers, which always seem to catch on something and so never stay closed long enough to heal.

If the cut gapes so badly that it cannot be held together with tape, or if it is deep enough to expose the layer of fat or muscle beneath the skin, it will need to be stitched. All cuts on the face, however minor, are best stitched to prevent scars.

Lacerations

A laceration is a tear in the skin and is usually caused by a hard blow or a serious injury. The skin edges are usually jagged, there is often considerable bruising around the wound, and infection is a particular hazard unless the wound is thoroughly cleaned.

Wounds of this sort will usually have to be seen by a doctor. They often bleed heavily and may be made worse by the

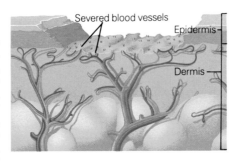

Abrasions are usually not as serious as they appear, though they may be very painful and leave scars afterwards. They must be thoroughly cleaned.

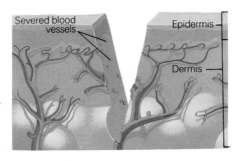

Cuts sometimes bleed profusely. They must be kept closed to heal properly and may need to be stitched, especially when they occur on the face.

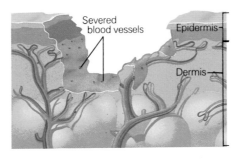

Lacerations are often serious wounds and take the longest time to heal. They should usually be seen by a doctor and kept covered meanwhile.

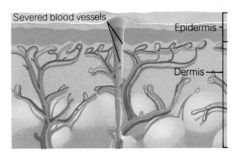

Puncture wounds are always more serious than they look, especially if to the abdomen or chest. Unless trivial, seek medical help as soon as possible.

presence of foreign objects like bullets or large splinters embedded in them. Never attempt to pull these out. They have already done all the damage they are going to do and trying to remove them may start off massive bleeding. You can stop them from working deeper into the wound by building up a thick 'ring' dressing around them, but leave anything more to the doctor. Bandage all lacerations with a large dressing until a doctor can treat the wound.

Puncture wounds

Finally, a puncture or stab wound is a small, deep wound of unknown depth caused, for example, when the prong of a garden fork is run through the foot.

It is most important that you do not try to stop the bleeding—this is the only way the wound can clean itself. Once the bleeding has stopped on its own, wash the wound and apply a clean, dry dressing.

Except for those made by something small and clean like a drawing pin, all puncture wounds require medical attention as there is danger of internal bleeding, damage to tendons and nerves and increased chance of infection and tetanus, as tetanus germs thrive in deep closed wounds, where there is no oxygen. A good rule of thumb is that a puncture or stab wound is always worse than it looks, so be sure to seek help for anything more than the most negligible wounds.

What the doctor will do

Although usually minor wounds will not need any medical attention, especially if first aid is applied quickly, major wounds or very dirty ones will need to be looked at by a doctor.

The doctor will clean the wound thoroughly and explore it to ensure that there are no remaining foreign bodies. If there is any risk that splinters of glass or bits of metal are still in the wound, an X-ray may be taken. The doctor will then check that the nerves and tendons are functioning normally and will decide whether a tetanus injection is necessary and whether the wound needs stitching (suturing).

Stitches are used to pull the edges of a gaping wound together. This closes the wound to further contamination, makes it easier for the edges to join together and decreases the chances of an unsightly scar. However, stitches will not be used if the wound can be held closed without them as they can injure the surrounding tissue slightly and may leave additional scars. To get the best result, stitching if it is needed should be done as soon as possible. A local anaesthetic will usually be given to deaden the area surrounding the wound.

Recognizing and treating serious wounds

FIRST AID

Aside from the specific wounds that require a doctor's attention, there are a few obvious signs that indicate that medical attention is needed urgently. Ideally one person should apply first aid while a second calls for help. If you are alone you will have to assess each situation individually and decide what immediate first aid is necessary before calling for help. All the instances below require medical attention, but this may only become apparent after initial first aid has been applied. Lose no time in seeking help when needed—never feel you should try to cope alone.

Symptoms	Possible causes	Action
Bleeding persists	An artery may have been severed, in which case the blood will spurt out with each heart beat. Or there may be a deep puncture	Apply pressure in the normal way for at least ten minutes. If an artery is severed try to locate a 'pressure point', a place where a main artery can be pressed against a bone. Pressure can be applied at these points to stop arterial blood loss, but it should not be applied for any longer than 15 minutes without a break
Patient shows signs of shock. Usually all the following symptoms will be present: pale face and lips, cold and clammy skin, faint or dizzy feeling and weak and rapid pulse	Caused by a combination of low blood pressure, constriction of blood vessels and blood loss. The body diverts remaining blood to essential organs, such as kidney, heart and brain. If shock is combined with no visible sign of blood loss, there may be internal bleeding	Place patient comfortably on side and cover with blankets or clothing. If possible, raise the feet so that blood is concentrated in the area of vital organs. Loosen any tight clothing. It is important to reassure someone in shock, so stay by the person if possible. Never give the patient any liquids
Patient experiences loss of movement or tingling sensations in the wounded area	A tendon or nerve may be severed (tendons attach muscles to the bone at joints, such as the knee)	Apart from general first aid, there is no immediate treatment for this. Try not to move the patient while awaiting medical help

Healing

Healing begins very soon after injury. The white blood cells that rush to the site of the wound to clear infection also remove any cells that have died as a result of the injury, as well as the small quantities of blood that have collected around the wound.

Once the injury is clean, the healing process can begin under the protective covering of the scab. The remaining live skin cells divide rapidly and begin to produce fibrous scar tissue, which contains blood vessels and nerve fibres. The scar tissue grows up from the base of the wound, gradually filling the hole. When this process has finished, the scab will fall off.

The more quickly the surfaces of a wound are brought together, either by stitching or bandaging, the less fibrous tissue is produced to bind them. Healing is therefore quicker and the wound leaves a fainter scar.

Wounds that have been stitched become waterproof within 24 hours and generally heal within five days, when the stitches can be removed. Over the next few months, all the reddish scar tissue becomes white as it gets denser and loses blood vessels. As the scar tissue becomes denser it contracts, and this causes the puckering that is sometimes seen around large scars. If a scar is unsightly it can be improved by a skin graft. Scar tissue never grows hairs, doesn't have sweat glands and will not turn brown in the sun, but it is strong and protects the body just as well as the original skin.

TAKE CARE

Wounds that require a doctor's attention

- wounds that will not stop bleeding
- any very large, deep, gaping or jagged wounds
- any wounds where dirt or grit are embedded beneath the skin
- puncture wounds caused by anything dirty or rusty
- any cut on the face
- any wound that shows signs of infection.

Even when the greatest care is taken with a wound, there is always a danger of infection developing. Local infection in a wound is quite common and will produce a discharge of pus. If the wound is relatively minor, the infection will probably be dealt with by the body's natural defence mechanisms, but if the area around the wounds becomes very red and irritated, or the patient develops a fever, a doctor should be consulted as antibiotics may be needed.

Any pus that is formed should be allowed to drain off. If the infected wound has been stitched, it may be necessary to release some of the stitches. Infected abrasions should be bathed and freshly dressed each day.

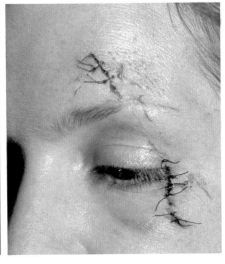

Ken Moreman

Abscess

Q If I have an abscess on a tooth, must I have the tooth out?

A Not necessarily. If you seek treatment early enough, the dentist can open the gum to drain the pus until the infection subsides, and can also prescribe antibiotics to prevent the infection from spreading. But often the only way to release the pus is by pulling out the tooth.

Q What is a gumboil?

A If infection gets in between the tooth and gum, a relatively harmless abscess will form, ballooning out the gum until it bursts. This gumboil is different to a dental abscess caused by infection in the tooth socket. A hot, salty mouthwash may relieve discomfort and help to rupture the abscess so that the pus can drain away, but if the trouble persists, visit the dentist.

Q How does all that pus get into an abscess?

A It doesn't actually 'get into' the abscess but builds up as part of the body's natural reaction to infection. Blood automatically rushes to the site of any injury, and when there is an infection the white blood cells, the body's infection-fighting team, move out of the damaged area into the infected tissue to kill the bacteria. In the struggle, the white blood cells often die themselves, and it is these dead cells, together with the dead bacteria, that form the well-known patch of yellow pus. At the same time, reserve forces of white blood cells build a wall that encloses the abscess's dangerous bacteria to keep the surrounding tissue intact and free from infection.

Q Why is an abscess in the ear so painful?

A Abscesses always involve considerable swelling. In the skin, this does not cause much discomfort, but in an area surrounded by bone, such as the ear, there is not enough space for this to happen without stretching the tissues around it, giving rise to great pain. For the same reason, severe discomfort accompanies any abscess in bone itself.

An abscess is the body's way of fighting localized infection. Minor abscesses often clear up with simple treatment, but larger or internal ones invariably need medical attention.

Abscesses can occur anywhere in, or on, the body. They range from simple styes, pimples and boils, which are abscesses in the skin's hair follicles, to serious tooth abscesses or other internal abscesses like appendicitis.

Causes
A skin abscess may result from an injury, such as a splinter, and is more likely to occur if damaged skin is dirty, or if the injury is in a moist area, such as the armpit, or if the person is run down.

Internal abscesses are usually secondary to some other problem—a 'grumbling appendix' may be caused by an internal abscess formed because an intestinal blockage has irritated the appendix—although, as with an abscess caused by tuberculosis, the disease-causing bacteria may be breathed in or ingested via contaminated food.

Symptoms
The earliest sign of a skin abscess is a red, hot, painful swelling, which becomes filled with pus. If white blood cells are able to cope with the bacteria, the abscess clears up without any discharge, becoming a hard, painless lump which may disappear after some months.

Other symptoms, particularly of internal abscesses, are a fever, feeling generally unwell and having swelling of the glands under the arms and elsewhere.

The great risk with an abscess is that on bursting it may release pus and dangerous live bacteria into the bloodstream, causing a serious type of blood-poisoning called septicaemia, or as in the case of an appendix abscess, into the abdominal cavity producing peritonitis (inflammation of the abdominal lining).

Treatment
Providing that a skin abscess is treated at an early stage and the pus is drained safely away, it will cause little more than discomfort. A small superficial abscess will often discharge pus of its own accord —or if obstinate, it can be 'lanced' with a sterile needle heated to red-hot and then allowed to cool. A touch of iodine or phenol will both sterilize and weaken the overlying skin, and applying magnesium sulphate paste on a *dry* dressing will help to draw out any remaining pus after the abscess has burst.

Large, deep abscesses need medical attention as the pus can only be safely drained by making an incision. Antiseptics and antibiotics will ensure that there is no danger of bacteria multiplying and spreading to healthy tissue.

Untreated tooth decay can sometimes cause an abscess. The obvious sign is severe toothache, and the tooth will be painful to bite on. The face may swell and an abscess may develop. If you get a tooth abscess, go to your dentist—it won't clear up by itself.

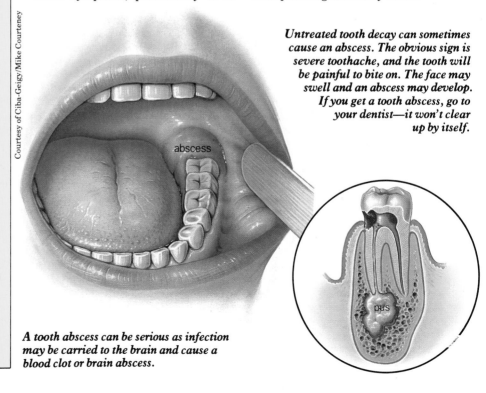

Courtesy of Ciba-Geigy/Mike Courteney

abscess

pus

A tooth abscess can be serious as infection may be carried to the brain and cause a blood clot or brain abscess.

Accident prevention

Q What can I do to help make sure that my children won't get injured at home?

A First make a safe house—then get into the right safety habits. Here are some of the most important points to keep in mind. Make sure that you NEVER . . .

● assume that visiting children have the same safety awareness as your own.
● allow children to play with sharp objects or run holding knives or scissors.
● permit games such as chasing on stairs or pushing wheeled toys into the kitchen.
● allow children to play with matches, lighters or cigarettes. Cigarette ends can poison a child.
● leave little ones in the bath alone.
● allow children to move electrical appliances alone, and never take any into the bathroom.
● leave baby alone with a bottle or young children with their meal. They could easily choke.
● allow young children to help with DIY jobs around the house.
● leave children alone with a hot iron while you go out of the room.
● keep medicines in your handbag. Never take them in front of the children or describe them as sweets.
● keep nursery goods such as gripe water in the same place as household goods like surgical spirit so that the two could get confused.
● leave plastic bags or polythene wrappers where the children can reach them and suffocate themselves.
● leave your child alone in the house even for five minutes.

Q Are there any particular times when my children are more likely to have accidents?

A Illness, tiredness, lack of supervision and general family stress may all make your child more prone to accidents. Weekends, when more is going on in the home, are a particularly hazardous time. Many injuries to children occur when their parents are either out of the house or asleep. Drugs can also contribute, so if, for example, your child is taking antihistamines for an allergy be especially watchful, as these medicines cause drowsiness.

Every year a large number of children have accidents in the home. Sadly, many die of their injuries. But most home accidents could easily be prevented if parents were more aware of the hazards—and made sure their home was safe for children.

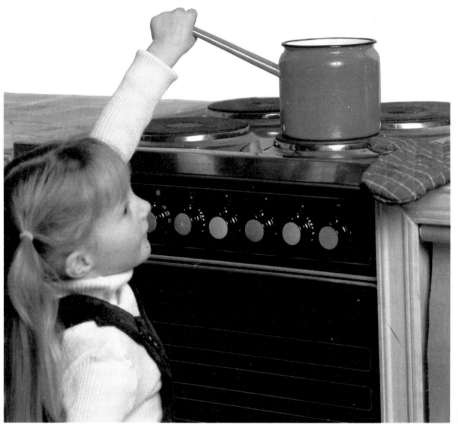

Di Lewis

Safety in the home is of the greatest importance for the well-being of children and parents alike. Recognizing the risks in the first place, and then taking adequate measures to ensure that your children are not in any danger is a vital part of responsible parenthood and will relieve you of much anxiety.

It is sensible to start making your home safe *before* you have a family so that when your children are born they start life in the best possible situation.

Preparing a safe home

If you are expecting a baby, start by drawing up a checklist of home safety measures you can carry out immediately. This should include making (or buying) safety gates for stairs, kitchen and outside doors; fixing loose rugs firmly to floors to avoid them causing falls; installing dummy plugs in any unused electric wall sockets; keeping dangerous household equipment out of children's reach— knives, can openers, cleaning powders; investing in safe heaters and fireguards; and ensuring that the home is well lit.

Next, learn safety habits yourself so that you will automatically follow them by the time you have children.

Lock away all medicines, including contraceptive pills and creams, indigestion tablets and iron and vitamin pills. Start running cold water before hot into the bath to avoid any danger of scalding at bathtime. Test out your furniture to discover which tables and chairs are least likely to topple over.

Take great care with fire and be especially careful in the kitchen, which is second only to the living/dining room as the most dangerous area in the house. If you do have a fire and cannot put it out easily, call the fire brigade. Make sure your older children know how to do this and keep your doctor's number by the telephone too.

Smooth areas of flooring in kitchens and bathrooms need non-slip surfaces like cork tiles, and liquid spills, especially of soap, cooking oil or other grease should be wiped up at once.

Day-to-day safety care

One of the commonest causes of death among the under-4s is suffocation—normally by choking on food—and the major cause of all hospital admissions for children under 14 is poisoning, either by medicines or by household substances. Among the 5s to 14s many deaths are from burns, while little ones aged one to two are vulnerable to all home accidents.

With a demanding baby, a safe daily routine will help when you are tired and preoccupied. Always put the things you use back in a safe place and do not use too much of anything—even talcum powder can cause choking. Be very watchful at bathtime. Do not be tempted to overfeed a baby, but if a baby does choke, keep calm and slap it between the shoulder blades to clear the air passages. After feeding always take the baby's bib off. Buy a cat net for the pram as cats are fond of seeking warmth from babies' blankets.

At the toddler stage—when children need particularly careful supervision—try to hear anything you cannot actually see, and beware of silence!

Clearly it is essential to supervise all meals. Spend time teaching your children how to climb stairs—they cause more accidents in the home than any other household objects—and show them how to balance and jump correctly from them. Help little ones to understand about hot and cold food and water, and show them how to carry breakable objects safely. Finally, to keep yourself alert, try to take some time off and hand the children over to someone you trust while staying on call should you be needed. The only common pets that are potentially dangerous are dogs. They should be obedience trained and never left alone with any child.

Children need careful supervision in the home, but at the same time it is important to allow them enough freedom to learn to deal independently and safely with their home environment.

Safe for children

Equipment bought especially for children is high on the danger list, but properly chosen, used and maintained it can be safe.

Prams should not tip over easily and should have an attachment for a safety harness. The brake should not be within the baby's reach and should work well even if the pram is tipped forward.

Folding pushchairs should have two sets of locking devices and so should the handle if this folds separately. Neither pushchairs nor prams can work properly if they are overloaded with other children or shopping.

Carry cots and stands should be sturdy and not easily tipped, and the handles should ensure a safe ride when the cot is carried by two people. If the cot is collapsible, it must not be likely to collapse accidentally. Ensure that the cot and stand are made of harmless rustproof material.

High chairs must be without sharp ends, open tubes where small limbs might get caught, or mechanisms that could pinch. The chair should not move on castors. Buy one that is at a convenient height, is sturdy, and has attachment points for a safety harness.

Night clothes must be flame-resistant, as should other clothes or the fabric you make them from.

Babies' clothes should be free from cords or other ties, which can interfere with circulation or could even hang or choke a baby.

Toddlers' clothes should allow freedom of movement and growth. They should be in at least part-natural fabric to allow the skin to breathe.

Toys are subject to government safety regulations in terms of materials used, instructions provided and the design and stability of larger items like baby walkers and tricycles. If a toy is secondhand, check it very carefully; some old toys were painted in a highly toxic lead paint. In general, wooden and plastic toys are safest. Never give a baby any toy that has removable buttons or bits that might be swallowed. All toys should be easy to clean.

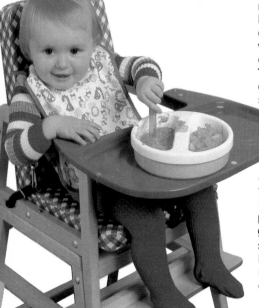

Di Lewis

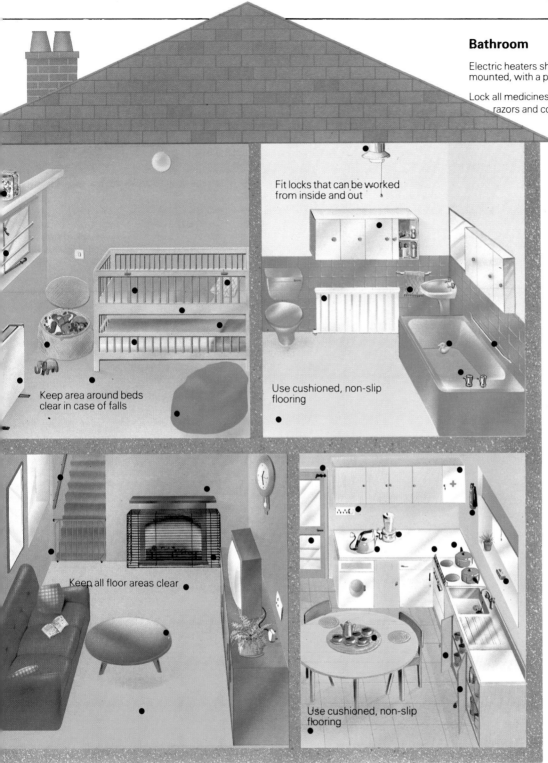

Fit locks that can be worked from inside and out

Keep area around beds clear in case of falls

Use cushioned, non-slip flooring

Keep all floor areas clear

Use cushioned, non-slip flooring

Bathroom

Electric heaters should be wall or ceiling mounted, with a pull switch at adult height

Lock all medicines in a cupboard. Put aerosols, razors and cosmetics in a high cupboard

Dry or air clothes over towel rails only

Radiators should not be too hot to touch. Keep hot water tank set at medium

Use large, preferably plastic bath toys

A hand grip and rubber mat prevent falls

Kitchen

Fit bolts to all doors that only adults can reach

Put matches well out of child's reach. Choose gas cooker without a pilot light and use an electric lighter

Keep a locked first aid box or cupboard to hand in kitchen

Keep a small fire extinguisher or heavy cloth near cooker to put out fires

Keep kettle and other electric equipment out of reach, on a short flex

Use tempered or laminated glass in doors, marked with tape or transfers so children don't walk into it

Ideally, fit a pan guard, or turn handles back out of reach

Use table mats instead of cloths. Keep hot drinks out of reach

Fit dummy plugs or covers on risky sockets

Put heavy items where they cannot fall on children

Leave only safe-to-play-with equipment in an unlocked floor-level cupboard

Put household cleaners in a locked cupboard or in a high place. Make sure they are clearly marked

---

Use absorbent cotton bed sheets (never plastic). Sheets should be fitted or lightly tucked in

Children's furniture should be soft, low and free from sharp edges, and positioned so that they cannot climb onto shelves or window sills

To prevent suffocation, use a porous type pillow, or none at all for babies under 1 year. Pillow cases should be cotton and well fitted

Living room

Fit a hand rail. Keep stairs well lit and free from ill-fitting carpets or jumble

An open fire must be fitted by law with a fixed guard. Position an extra one far enough away so that the bars do not get hot

Keep area over fire clear to avoid attracting a child's attention

Use safety gates, at top and bottom of stairs, at kitchen doors and other potentially dangerous places

Make sure all furniture and fitments are secure and will support a child's weight

Ideally, fit a hard-wearing carpet except in kitchen and bath. Or fix any loose rugs to prevent slips. Do not lay rugs on polished floors

Acne

Q Does acne always leave scars on the skin?

A No, but the chances of scarring are increased if you pick and squeeze the spots. However, even if the blackheads are not squeezed, scars may still form. If they are severe they can be partially removed by a minor surgical operation called dermabrasion, in which the top layers of skin are rubbed away, leaving the skin relatively smooth.

Q My daughter has very bad acne. Should I take her to the doctor?

A Yes. The doctor can prescribe antibiotics over a period of several months to reduce secondary infection of the spots by bacteria, or may put her on the birth control Pill, which contains hormones that help correct the hormone imbalance that causes acne. And the reassurance and advice about hygiene the doctor gives may well be easier for your daughter to accept as it comes from someone outside the family circle.

Q Is it true that chocolate causes acne?

A Acne has several causes that are not necessarily connected with diet. It is was once thought that cutting out chocolate would help it clear up more quickly and stop new spots forming. There is no certainty, however, that chocolate is the culprit but if you have acne, it may be worth dropping it from your diet for a while to see whether it makes any difference. There are several other foods which sometimes affect acne, and your doctor may suggest that you try avoiding them too. On the positive side, he may suggest you eat lots of fresh fruit and vegetables and drink plenty of water.

Q I get the occasional spot. Is this acne?

A No, acne is a whole mass of blackheads and pimples. The odd spot can also be caused by a hormone imbalance, as before a period, but it is just as likely that an unhealthy diet, poor hygiene or being run down is to blame.

The pimpled face of adolescence is so common that it could almost be thought of as normal. Four out of five teenagers suffer from acne to some degree, but the majority grow out of it. In the meantime, there are preventive measures and treatments which can ease the problem.

The mixture of blackheads, whiteheads and pink or reddish spots caused by *Acne vulgaris* occurs mostly on the face, the back of the neck, the upper back and chest, but can sometimes be found in the armpits and on the buttocks, too.

Causes

Acne affects young people of both sexes but tends to be more common in boys. It starts in adolescence because this is when there are great increases in the production of hormones from the sex organs and from the adrenal glands. These hormones are chemical messengers carried by the blood and transform a child into a sexually mature adult.

Under their influence, and particularly that of the androgens, or 'masculinizing'

hormones, the oil-releasing sebaceous glands in the skin, which normally produce just enough oil or sebum to keep the skin healthily supple, become overactive. They release too much sebum, causing a condition called *seborrhoea*.

The female hormones, particularly oestrogen, have the reverse effect, which explains—at least in part—why girls are generally less prone to acne than boys.

Symptoms

Blackheads, accompanied by the pink or reddish inflammation which they cause, are the hallmark of acne. It was once thought that the bacteria that naturally thrive on sebum, particularly two called *Staphylococcus albus* and *Bacillus acnus,* were the underlying cause of the acne,

How to alleviate the symptoms of acne

AVOID
- greasy hair oils or cosmetics.
- leaving makeup on overnight—or leave it off completely
- applying creams to dirty skin so that bacteria are pushed into the pores
- eating any foods that seem to cause spots

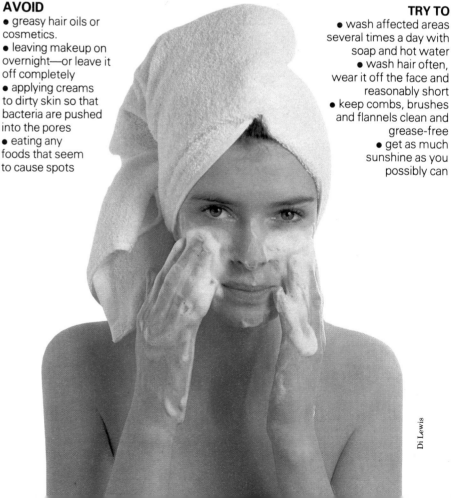

TRY TO
- wash affected areas several times a day with soap and hot water
- wash hair often, wear it off the face and reasonably short
- keep combs, brushes and flannels clean and grease-free
- get as much sunshine as you possibly can

Di Lewis

but they are now known to be the cause of the inflammation, not the acne itself.

In response to the presence of bacteria, which multiply in the blackhead, the blood vessels expand to bring more infection-fighting cells to the site—this is the inflammatory reaction. As a secondary effect of acne, the bacterial infection may lead to the development of pimples, which are spots filled with dead white cells and bacteria, or pus.

This infection usually only becomes severe, involving the formation of larger boils or abscesses, if the deeper skin tissues become bruised and damage as a result of squeezing the blackheads to release the core of sebum plugged in the pore. Left undisturbed, each spot or blackhead usually clears up within about a week, but if secondary infection sets in it may take a month or more.

Dangers

Secondary infection is one of the chief physical dangers of acne, as it can lead to severe permanent scars and crater-like pits of pock-marks in the complexion. Even more severe is the psychological danger, for acne can return a happy extrovert into a morose introvert. So anyone suffering from acne needs all the reassurance possible to prevent a temporary physical problem from becoming one that is psychologically permanent.

Try to take a practical approach to treatment and dispel any fears engendered by old wives' tales—for example, that acne is caused by masturbation or sexual intercourse.

Treatment

On a day-to-day basis, the most important treatment is washing. This is most effective if it is as vigorous as possible,

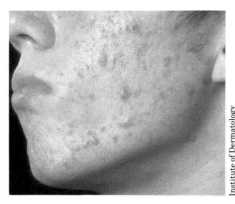

Institute of Dermatology

and a soft nailbrush or loofah—kept scrupulously clean to avoid reinfection—will help to remove grease and encourage the top layer of skin to peel away, taking with it some, if not all, of the plug of sebum. Drying, equally vigorously, with a rough, clean towel will have the same effect. An astringent cleansing lotion applied with clean cotton wool after thorough washing will help to remove any remaining oil.

It is possible to remove the blackheads with an instrument called a comedone extractor. However, this must be used with great care, preferably only on the recommendation of a doctor, and with meticulous attention to hygiene, to prevent the possibility of secondary infection.

A clean face will be of little help to the acne problem if it is then surrounded by lank, greasy hair. Unfortunately the overactivity of the sebaceous glands is not confined to the face but also affects the scalp, and the hair tends to become excessively greasy with the usual associated development of scurf or dandruff. The grease from the hair aggravates the acne, so hair should be washed regularly and kept reasonably short.

Creams and lotions can be useful to treat acne, as much for their camouflage effect as for medical reasons. The best preparations are those that contain substances such as calamine, zinc sulphate, sulphur, resorcinol or benzoyl peroxide, which tend to dry the skin and cause peeling of the top layer. Boys may regard such creams as an insult to their masculinity, but many modern ones are very natural-looking and may prove a very useful psychological prop.

A well balanced diet containing plenty of fresh fruit and vegetables is always good for the skin, and the acne sufferer is advised to drink a lot of water to keep the circulation well flushed of the toxins that are likely to aggravate the condition.

Many acne sufferers find that spots clear up more quckly in summer. This is because the ultra-violet light in sunshine helps dry up grease on the skin and aids peeling of the top layer. For the same reason, ultra-violet ray lamps are often advised for acne sufferers, but these should be used with care to prevent the skin burning.

It is always sensible for a teenager with very bad acne to see a doctor, who may be able to prescribe treatment not available over the chemist's counter.

Outlook

The best that can be said for acne is that it does not last forever. Usually there is only one really bad year, and acne is rare after the mid-twenties. Difficult though it may be to follow, the best advice is to resist with a will of iron the temptation to pick and squeeze blackheads.

Finally, keep a look out for new treatments, such as preparations containing retinoic acid, which have shown encouraging results in clinical trials.

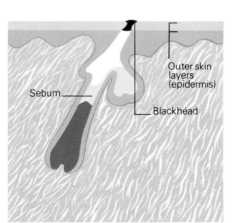

In acne, extra sebum (oil) first clogs up the pores through which sebum is released to the skin surface.

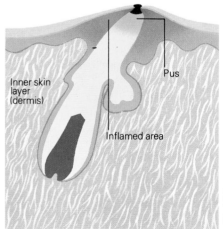

Nigel Osborne

The sebum is trapped and forms a plug with a raised top which, when exposed to air, becomes a blackhead.

The surrounding skin then becomes inflamed and infected, resulting in pimples filled with pus.

Acupuncture

Q Will acupuncture help me to stop smoking?

A Only if you really want to stop. It will help by reducing the withdrawal symptoms and the craving.

Q I've seen pictures of people with acupuncture needles in them. It looks as though it might be painful.

A Most people experience very little discomfort. There is a slight, brief prick as the needle enters the skin, but as the treatment takes effect there is usually a feeling of numbness, aching, swelling or tingling.

Q Does the insertion of the needles make you bleed?

A Usually no, because the smooth, fine and supple needles do not damage the tissues. Points on the ear and face bleed occasionally as the skin here has a rich blood supply.

Q How long does the treatment take to work?

A This depends on several factors. Acute complaints may improve immediately or within a week or two. Chronic conditions will take longer, perhaps two or three months of weekly treatments, although some benefit should be noticed within a few weeks.

Q Do I need a referral from my doctor before visiting an acupuncturist?

A A referral is not necessary, although it is always appreciated. If there is a good reason for you not to have acupuncture, your doctor will explain this to you.

Q Can people of all ages receive acupuncture?

A As a rough guide, anyone between the ages of 7 and 70 can receive acupuncture. If a child is not afraid of needle pricks and can remain still then there should be no problem. With older patients, moxibustion is often preferred to needle treatment.

Cure-all or con trick? Today, an increasing number of people are turning to acupuncture, and though not a miracle remedy, it does offer an alternative method of relieving pain and modern stress-related complaints.

Acupuncture is an ancient healing art that has been used in China for several thousand years. Following the discovery of acupuncture anaesthesia in China during the 1950s, several groups of Western doctors visited China to report on the technique. They were impressed, and interest in acupuncture grew rapidly with many of the techniques being incorporated into Western medical practice. Although often regarded as an alternative medicine, it has been surprisingly successful in the treatment of many ailments where more conventional methods have failed.

Perhaps the failure of acupuncture to become fully integrated with Western medical practice is due to the great difference between the cultures of the East and West. In ancient China, the emphasis was on preventative medicine, something which is relatively new in Western medical thought. It is this cultural division that has produced two explanations of how acupuncture works.

The Chinese origins

Acupuncture has its roots in the ancient Chinese philosophy of Taoism, where it was believed that man is one with the universe and that all life is permeated with the life-giving energy of Chi. Part of this belief is that all our experiences have opposites (hot/cold, day/night, masculine/feminine). Yin and Yang are the names given to these opposite forces.

The theory is that Yin and Yang merge and complement one another, creating a balance. When the forces are balanced we are in good health. However, when the flow is out of balance within ourselves and with the universe we feel unwell and disease may develop.

Acupuncture is used to restore the balance, the acupuncture points being the places where treatment is applied. These acupuncture points lie above lines under the skin called meridians, and the ancient theorists believed these lines acted as channels through which the Yin and Yang energies flowed. Whether one is sympathetic to this theory or not, acupuncture worked for the ancient Chinese.

Modern theory

Today, Western practitioners of acupuncture explain its effectiveness in more scientific terms, though still incorporating some of the Oriental beliefs.

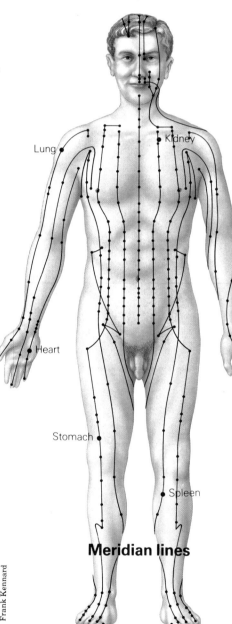

Lung

Kidney

Heart

Stomach

Spleen

Frank Kennard

Meridian lines

Their explanation is based on Western knowledge of the body's nervous system.

Beneath the skin is a widespread network of nerves, the most important strands of which run along the meridians where most acupuncture points lie.

Among their functions, the nerves pass on messages that take the form of feelings which tell us what state our bodies are in. These messages come from all over the body and when they arrive from a damaged organ an 'alarm' sounds at the

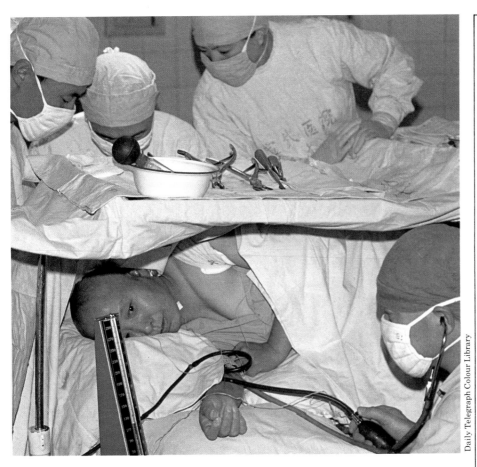

Daily Telegraph Colour Library

nerve endings in the skin. When this happens the alarm is felt as pain. The theory is that the pain may be referred; that is, it may be a signal of a problem located elsewhere in the body rather than where the pain is felt.

For instance, pain from the stomach is registered in the skin of the upper abdomen and the adjacent part of the back. The connection between the source of the problem and where the pain is felt is explained by the fact that both areas have interconnecting nerves.

There are a thousand or so acupuncture points in the body dotted along the meridian lines. There are 12 main meridians and each is associated with an organ of the body. The lines run along the major parts of the body (such as the arms and legs) and end at the tips of the fingers or the toes. For instance, the liver meridian runs down the inside of the left leg, from the midriff to the big toe.

How it works
Although the ancient Chinese believed that it was the rebalancing of Yin and Yang energies that brought relief, modern scientific studies have indicated that there are at least two alternative theories.

The 'gate theory' is that there are reflex mechanisms in the nerve pathways

Acupuncture needles can be inserted in any of the thousand or so points along the meridian lines. The needles have an anaesthetic effect powerful enough to allow brain surgery to take place with the patient fully conscious.

which can close off pain, rather as if a gate were being closed. This reduces the pain although the cause persists. Acupuncture works by closing these gates.

The other theory explains the success of acupuncture through the production of hormones called endorphins. These have a pain-killing effect, much like the drug morphine. There is now evidence that acupuncture causes the release of endorphins and these then travel to the brain, where they activate a mechanism which blocks the pain messages.

This theory helps to explain the pain-relieving effects of acupuncture and its ability to induce relaxation and a sense of well-being. However, no theory as yet manages to explain some of the claims of wonder cures.

The benefits of acupuncture
Acupuncture can be used to help with a wide range of specific problems, not just the relief of pain. These include headaches, rheumatic pains, digestive disorders, asthma, hypertension, insomnia,

anxiety, menstrual disorders and infertility. It is also used in childbirth and even in open-heart operations.

The treatment also gives a feeling of well-being and relaxation. For this reason it is an appropriate treatment or preventive for the numerous ailments caused by stress in our high-speed society. But acupuncture is not a cure-all. It is not appropriate for anyone who is at risk from infection (i.e. severe diabetics or people taking steroids), nor for those who have bleeding disorders such as haemophilia.

Treatment
The patient is questioned about his complaint and asked whether diet, mood, personal habits, season and weather have any effect on the problem.

A thorough physical examination then takes place, with the acupuncturist taking particular note of any tender areas, the pulse rate at the wrist, signs of tension, and variations in body temperature. Further information is sometimes obtained from examining the tongue, iris, and soles of the feet.

For pain relief in childbirth, needles may be inserted in the toe, earlobe and hand. Those in the hand may be electrically stimulated according to the strength of the contractions. Only a slight tingling sensation is felt.

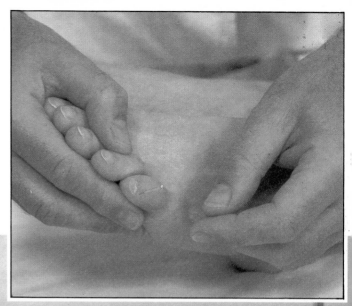

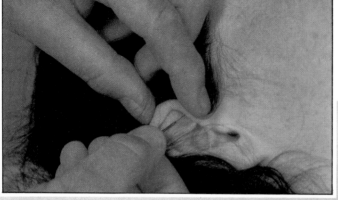

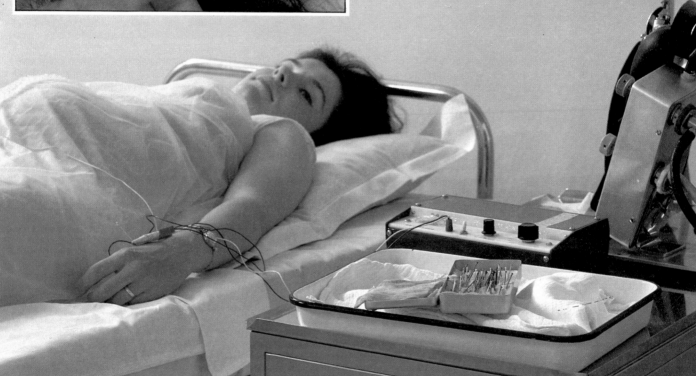

On the basis of all this information a diagnosis can be made, either in terms of diseases or of the classical concepts of Chi energy balance. The treatment then consists of applying needles, massage or heat to certain points on the body.

The heat treatment is called moxibustion because it involves placing rolled-up cones of the herb moxa on the correct meridian points and igniting them. A beneficial warmth is produced by their slow burning and the acupuncturist removes them before the skin is reached. Heat treatment can also be provided by electrical means, using a recent Japanese invention, but acupuncturists generally consider that it is no substitute for the original method.

The choice of the points depends on the condition of the patient; it will vary from person to person and from day to day as the condition changes. The number of needles used also changes; from one to 20 or more, and they may stay in for as long as the acupuncturist deems necessary.

The success of the treatment depends on many factors, among them diet and lifestyle.

One risk involved is that acupuncture applied thoughtlessly might hide a serious illness by taking away the symptoms. This is the reason for the very thorough examination and diagnosis.

A common response to the treatment is that the patients become so relaxed that they temporarily lose co-ordination after

a session. For this reason, alcohol and sedatives should not be combined with acupuncture. Driving is also unwise, especially after the first session.

Treatment at home

Some acupuncture techniques can be learnt and practised at home. This applies more to acupressure, which is a form of massage acupuncture without needles. It will provide relief from headaches, tension and anxiety, among other stress complaints, and is perfectly safe. The use of acupuncture is growing rapidly. There are now many colleges that provide training in acupuncture and acupressure for those who wish to become qualified practitioners.

Adenoids

Q My child breathes through his mouth a lot. Does this mean he has adenoid trouble?

A Not necessarily. But if he also has nasal discharge and a night-time cough, adenoids are probably the cause. Otherwise it may be a habit, and is best cured by regular noseblowing. You should check his ability to breathe through each nostril in turn to make sure that something lodged in the nose is not the cause. A few children are born with bone abnormalities which prevent normal nose-breathing.

Q Can adenoids be diagnosed just by looking at a child's face?

A No. So-called 'adenoidal faces' have been found to occur in many other conditions. The description refers to a snub nose, high arched palate and protruberant upper teeth, which give the child a rather dopey look.

Q If my child has had his adenoids operated on can they regrow?

A Yes. They can regrow because it is surgically impossible to remove the whole of the glands. They are merely cut off as low as possible. This leaves a small stump which can enlarge again. However, as the stimulus to grow disappears around the age of six, regrowth does not usually cause problems.

Q How long is it safe to use decongestant nosedrops?

A Any runny nose will be dried up by decongestant drops. The problem is that if the cause has not been dealt with, stopping the drops will cause the discharge to return. In the case of adenoids, the problem for which they are needed will probably have improved after a week or so, and they should be stopped then. A slight discharge may return for a day or two, which will have to be tolerated without restarting the drops. If the drops are used for more than three weeks continually, there is a definite risk that the nose will counterbalance their effect by running all the time. And prolonged use can cause serious damage.

The adenoids have been called 'the watchdogs of the throat'. Like the tonsils, they guard against respiratory infection in the young child, but like the tonsils they sometimes become infected and swollen themselves.

Adenoids are lymph glands situated at the back of the nose just where the air passages join those of the back of the mouth or pharynx. The lymph system is the body's defence against infection and the lymph glands, such as the adenoids, are full of infection-fighting cells, the white blood cells. The adenoids are so placed that any infection breathed in through the nose is filtered by them and—hopefully—killed. Sometimes, however, things can go wrong.

Causes
Adenoids are present from birth, but on the whole they disappear before puberty. They are most obvious from the age of one to four. This is because between these ages the child is continually exposed to new types of infection.

Inflamed and swollen adenoids can block the Eustachian tubes and lead to ear infections and even deafness.

Not a great deal is known about how the adenoids become infected, but any respiratory germ can affect them. Once they become damaged, chronic infection may set in. If the adenoids are recurrently inflamed, they tend to swell and this can give rise to ill-effects.

Symptoms
If the glands become swollen due to infection, they interfere with the flow of air through the nose so that the child has to breathe through the mouth. This may cause heavy snoring at night. The closed mouth also causes a nasal tone of speech. The child finds that his 'm' comes out as 'b' and 'n' sounds like 'd'. This is because when he closes his mouth to pronounce 'm' and 'n' through the nose, he cannot do so since his nose is blocked. Breathing

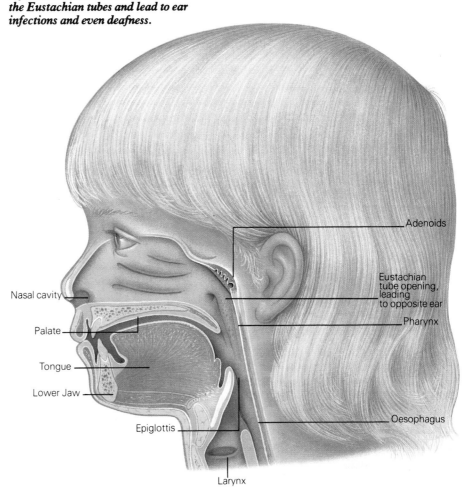

Nasal cavity

Palate

Tongue

Lower Jaw

Epiglottis

Larynx

Adenoids

Eustachian tube opening, leading to opposite ear

Pharynx

Oesophagus

Mike Courteney

Q Is sneezing and a runny nose due to adenoids?

A Usually not. These symptoms are more suggestive of an allergic nose problem. As research continues, many childhood illnesses are being found to be due to allergies. Often these are caused by dusts and pollens, and sneezing or a runny nose is their most obvious symptom. The medical treatment with decongestants and antihistamines is the same, but adenoidectomy would make no difference.

Q Is there a link between adenoids and mental deficiency?

A Certainly not! Though children with an adenoid problem may look dull and be slow to respond, careful studies have failed to show any such link. However, if left completely untreated, the complication of deafness can certainly prevent a child from realizing his true potential.

Q My child snores heavily. Could he have adenoids?

A Snoring can certainly be due to enlarged adenoids, but by itself this symptom does not need treating. Otherwise, snoring could be caused by an abnormality of the facial structure which the child probably had since birth. Many children breathe noisily at night, which is not true snoring but just a result of a catarrhal complaint such as the common cold.

Q Can antihistamines and antibiotics do anything to help treat adenoids?

A Antihistamines reduce the swelling of the adenoids when this has been caused by an allergic reaction as opposed to infection, and they will also tend to reduce the discharge as well. A further benefit is that antihistamines usually cause drowsiness and combat nausea so a bedtime dose will reduce coughing and the morning vomiting.

Antibiotics are of benefit for enlarged adenoids only when there is also a bacterial infection and must be prescribed by your doctor. The adenoidal symptoms may remain but painful complications such as ear infections can be prevented.

through the mouth also makes it very dry and the child may continually ask for something to drink.

As the adenoids fight infection, white blood cells—both dead and alive—are released in the form of pus. This pus will be seen as a discharge from the nose— quite different from the clear, watery discharge of a runny cold. The child sniffs to try to clear it but it then runs down the back of his throat and makes him cough. The cough is particularly obvious at night and is a typical sign of infected adenoids. In the morning, the swallowed pus may cause vomiting.

Dangers
Swollen adenoids can block the Eustachian tubes, which are a pair of tunnels running through the skull bones from inside each eardrum to the pharynx. Their function is to equalize the pressure in the middle ears with that outside— they give rise to the familiar 'pop' you hear on swallowing. If the tube is blocked by the enlarged adenoids the pressure cannot be balanced.

But the main hazard is that natural secretions in the ear cannot drain from inside. This gives rise to a 'glue ear' in which the hearing apparatus is stuck up by secretions and hearing is impaired.

And the secretions themselves may become infected causing a condition called *otitis media*. This is painful and can affect the hearing permanently. If untreated, the eardrums will usually burst to release the infection.

Treatment
Gargling is useless, but three types of medicines are helpful in treating adenoids. Decongestants and antihistamines are on sale at the chemist, but consult your doctor before using them. Antibiotics are available only on prescription.

As a last resort, when other methods have failed, the adenoids may be removed by an operation called an adenoidectomy. The operation is fairly simple and is carried out under a general anaesthetic in hospital. The tonsils are often removed in the same operation.

Outlook
Providing none of the serious complications occur, time, the decline of infectious diseases and improvements in treatment all mean that adenoids are not the problem they were twenty years ago. Often symptoms go away of their own accord when the child is six or so, and modern medicines usually save small children from an operation.

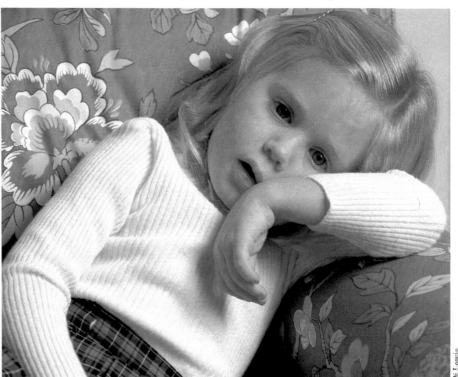

Some common symptoms of swollen adenoids

- hearing difficulties
- dry gums, which result in tooth decay, and halitosis
- loss of smell, taste and appetite
- listless expression, because breathing is such hard work

Adolescence

Q We used to have a very close relationship with our son. Now he has turned completely against us. Where did we go wrong?

A Nowhere. It is often the case that the closer the relationship, the more sudden the rebellion in adolescence. Just remember that this does not mean rejection. A child who storms at his or her parents still obviously cares what they think—more so probably than a child who simply ignores them.

Q Our 16-year-old daughter wants to go on the Pill, although she swears she is not sleeping with anyone. She says it is 'just in case'. Should I let her?

A Although you may be worried, the fact that she has consulted you is a compliment to your relationship with her. But do not forbid her to go on the Pill; she could consult a doctor and it would be prescribed if it was thought that she was sufficiently mature and responsible. You would not be told because medical matters are always confidential. Remember also that preventing her from going on the Pill will not stop her from having sexual relationships. So be realistic—she could come to you in a couple of months' time wanting not the Pill but an abortion. Or not coming to you at all, which would be worse.

Talk to her calmly and sympathetically. Point out that the Pill is a drug which should not be taken unnecessarily. Tell her what you feel, but remember that she needs to make her own decision once she is armed with a range of opinions and as much factual information as possible.

Q My 15-year-old son is terribly rude to me and my husband, but I'm afraid if I put my foot down it will turn him against us.

A Do put your foot down—firmly. In the long run, he'll respect you for it, and that means you'll be doing him a favour: children who have no regard for their parents often never develop any self-respect themselves.

In adolescence young people are undergoing the physical and mental changes that take them into adulthood, and this can be a difficult time for them. It is vital that parents show sympathy and understanding—and are able to judge when professional help is needed.

Adolescence begins with the onset of puberty, when the body begins to develop rapidly. Boys quickly grow taller and more muscular at an amazing speed. Girls, too, increase rapidly in height; body fat begins to be redistributed to breasts, buttocks, hips and thighs and the menstrual periods start. In boys, the penis and testicles grow larger. Both sexes develop body hair in the armpits, the groin and on the limbs; boys begin to grow facial hair.

These changes are brought about by a complex interplay of hormones, or 'chemical messengers'—which are released into the bloodstream by the glands. Their effect is not only physical but also mental and emotional.

On average, adolescence starts around the age of 11 for girls and 13 for boys, but it can in fact begin at any time from 10 to 16 in both sexes.

A time of conflict

Before adolescence, girls mature physically and mentally about two years ahead of boys; but then boys seem to overtake them in academic ambition and physical prowess, while most girls adopt a passive role in keeping with the expectations of society. Yet both sexes share a surging physical, emotional and mental strength, coupled with a powerful sexual drive and a growing sense of independence and individuality.

Since it is generally true that these characteristics are encouraged in boys and suppressed in girls, both sexes can feel a great sense of conflict. Girls who want to compete in a man's world may not be encouraged to do so, then may indulge

A feeling of independence will prompt many adolescents to venture out into the world to earn their own money.

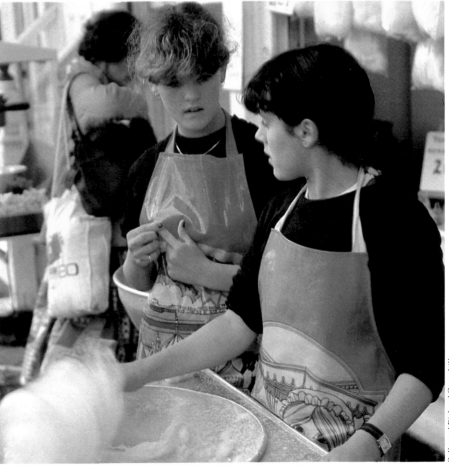

Sally and Richard Greenhill

Q Our eldest daughter was nothing but trouble all the time she was in her teens. But our second girl is as quiet as a mouse and doesn't give us a moment's worry. Is this significant?

A Not really. The amount of trouble children are in adolescence isn't necessarily an indication of how they will behave in adult life.

Parents often worry about their first child. This is mainly because they are adjusting to the responsibilities of parenthood and so the child may be under pressures which make him or her react strongly. A younger child is not under so much pressure and so is likely to behave differently. But if you think your second daughter is too quiet, you should seek advice from a professional counsellor.

Q I found a collection of dirty magazines under my son's bed. What should I do?

A Adolescents tend to be pre-occupied with sex. All you need to do is to point out that they offend *you* and that you would rather he did not leave them where you can find them. If you make too much of a fuss they could take on the attraction of forbidden fruit.

But what are you doing looking under his bed in the first place? After all, they were out of sight. It sounds as though he's more considerate of you than you are of him—and is probably more able to handle 'adult' thoughts than you give him credit for.

Q My teenager has begun to ask me the most bizarre questions about God, the meaning of life, and so forth. Is this normal?

A Yes, in fact it's probably the sign of a lively, enquiring mind grappling with some of the fundamental questions of life. Adolescence is a period when growing children begin to be fascinated by obscure and often seemingly pointless questions—and impatient with adults who, having become adjusted to the existence of death, whether or not there is a God, or the state of the world, show little interest in discussing these matters. But they can be of profound interest to adolescents, who are aware of them as topics for the first time.

in rebellious behaviour; boys who display sensitivity and many of the caring traits encouraged in girls often have trouble relating to both sexes, who are brought up to expect 'masculine' behaviour in boys.

Young men have just as difficult a time in many ways as girls. Not only are they expected to be 'strong', both physically and in their support of the opposite (and supposedly weaker) sex, but they are also expected to be successful providers. This can place a great burden on the male adolescent who may be frightened of failure in both respects, and this may cause him to revert to child-like behaviour when under stress.

Contradictory and confused behaviour can worry and annoy parents, who have perhaps forgotten that they went through exactly the same turmoil. It needs great patience to cope with an individual who demands to be treated as an adult one minute and then throws a fit of temper or demands help, support and reassurance, just like a child, the next.

How can parents help?

The most important thing that parents can do to help adolescent children is to become less obviously their protectors and disciplinarians, while still remaining a 'safety net' should problems arise.

Obviously, this change has to take place over a period of time, ending when the children have reached a recognized state of adulthood and feel they are ready to leave home and fend for themselves.

Though they are reluctant to admit it, adolescents really do rely very much on their parents. This is the time of life when they are trying to work things out for themselves, but they still need someone to turn to for support when a situation becomes too difficult for them to cope with.

What is 'normal' behaviour?

Sometimes the various kinds of experimentation or rebellion in which adolescents may become involved can get out of control, yet the children will not admit anything to their parents. How can you tell if things have got out of hand?

The mental state of adolescents is often very confusing to an outsider. The parental cry most often heard by doctors is, 'I'm sure he—or she—isn't normal . . .'

Moodiness, an entirely normal—but usually temporary—stage, can result in the adoption of unconventional or outlandish points of view, and these can also be very disturbing. In the main, there is no great significance in this stage of mental development, although it may seem at times morbid for a healthy youngster to be preoccupied with death or religion, or just pure obstinacy for a

Normal behaviour in adolescence

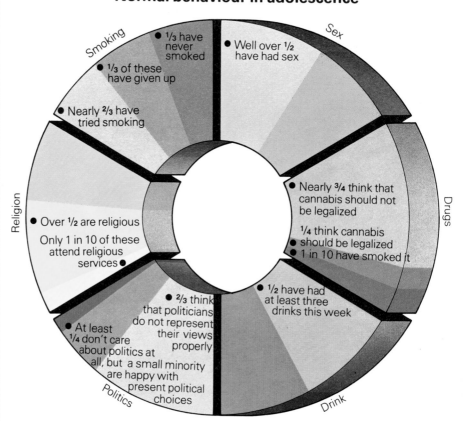

- **Smoking** — 1/3 have never smoked
- 1/3 of these have given up
- Nearly 2/3 have tried smoking
- **Sex** — Well over 1/2 have had sex
- **Drugs** — Nearly 3/4 think that cannabis should not be legalized
- 1/4 think cannabis should be legalized
- 1 in 10 have smoked it
- **Religion** — Over 1/2 are religious. Only 1 in 10 of these attend religious services
- 1/2 have had at least three drinks this week
- 2/3 think that politicians do not represent their views properly
- At least 1/4 don't care about politics at all, but a small minority are happy with present political choices
- **Politics**
- **Drink**

teenager to hold forth noisily on left or right-wing politics to parents who are of the opposite persuasion.

Danger signals

The most common problem in adolescence is depression. This can be either a reaction to some event—such as the failure of an important examination, the inability to find a job, the loss of a boy or girl friend—or can simply 'come from within' happening for no apparent external reason. The symptom is always deep apathy. The young person shows no interest in anything, is listless, uncommunicative and mopes about. Sleeping habits are disturbed, he or she may wake early in the morning, continue to lie awake, and then stay in bed complaining of tiredness long after everyone else is up.

Unfortunately, there is an increasing trend of teenage depression leading to suicide—or attempted suicide. It is vital to watch for danger signals such as deep introspection, furtive behaviour, drinking or outbursts of aggression and violence. Do not try to play amateur psychiatrist or put a label on why a child seems depressed. If there appears to be any cause for concern or anxiety, ask for outside help. It is far better to play safe than be sorry.

Drug abuse is sometimes a worry to parents of adolescent children, but there

Adolescents often feel out of tune with the rest of society and form close friendships with their equals.

are two reassuring factors which should be borne in mind: firstly, drug use among teenagers is decreasing; secondly, an isolated incident of smoking cannabis is unlikely to do much harm.

However, evidence of using stimulants, such as amphetamines or 'speed', should be viewed with concern. But it is the 'hard' drugs—like heroin and morphine —that are potential killers.

Another disturbing trend is 'glue sniffing'. Unfortunately the glue is cheap, readily available—and lethal. Prompt medical treatment, combined with social counselling, is essential in all these cases.

As drug-taking declines among teenagers, so the use of alcohol increases. They may pick up the habit from parents, or drink simply because they know their parents would disapprove. This may appear to be a contradiction, but is typical of much adolescent behaviour.

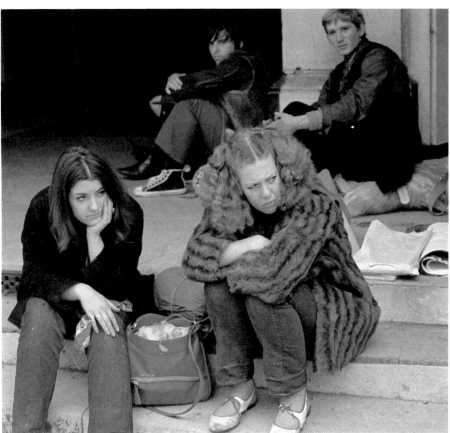

Rex Features

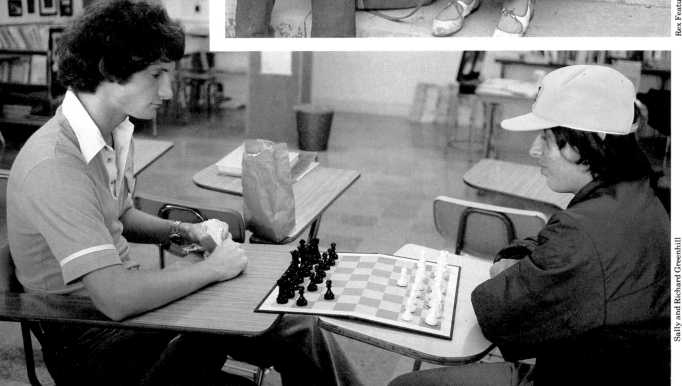

Sally and Richard Greenhill

Social problems

Rowdiness and vandalism cause great concern both to parents and the general public. Unfortunately, such anti-social activities can be part of growing up and proving independence. The adolescent, having rejected the security of the home but not yet ready to take on the adult world, finds security in a group of friends who have devised their own rules about dress and conduct.

Groups such as skinheads, rockers or punks are bound by strong ties within and hostility to other groups, which can, in extreme cases, erupt in gang warfare. But those who become involved in serious violence more often than not come from violent or deprived homes and so adolescence is not necessarily the root cause.

Sexual problems

To adolescents themselves, sex poses perhaps the biggest problem of all. Many are confused by their awakening sexual instincts and some may react either by becoming introspective and shy or by behaving outrageously. They need time to adjust their self-image to include this new aspect to their lives.

An important part of their development will be a growing interest in the opposite sex. Dating, going out and getting to know a number of different boyfriends or girlfriends is the way they learn to relate to people in adult life.

Part of any relationship with the opposite sex will invariably involve some sexual experimentation, as both sexes explore their own and each other's physical and emotional responses to sex.

There is, of course, no guaranteed formula that parents can adopt to ensure that teenagers do not find themselves involved in premature sexual relationships. But good sex education both at home and at school may be a way of ensuring that adolescents do understand about sex, responsibility and birth control. This means that parents and teachers need to be sympathetic, sensitive and able to discuss sexuality in a straightforward and caring manner.

Another worry for parents may be that their child will become a homosexual, especially if he or she is not interested in the opposite sex. But at this stage in life, it is entirely normal for young people to enjoy close relationships with others of their own sex and this does not mean that they will be homosexual in adult life.

Setting an example

The way parents themselves behave can be crucial in dealing with adolescent problems. The example they set their children is far more important than giving them moral lectures. If they show sympathy and understanding, and make constant efforts to communicate, they will give their children the best chance of overcoming adolescent problems and becoming well-adjusted adults.

Problems which may affect adolescents

Problems	Reasons	Signs	How parents should react
Depressed behaviour	Inability to make friends; school or exam problems; loss of boyfriend/girlfriend; bad self-image; anxiety about the state of the world; no apparent reason	Apathy; introspection; secrecy; tiredness; bad schoolwork; disturbed sleep; surliness; difficulty in communicating or refusal to communicate at all; threats of suicide	Consult the school as to the situation; ask advice from family doctor or psychologist; bolster child's self-esteem in terms of appearance and ego; never shout 'Snap out of it!'; ask yourself: are you expecting too much? Are you caring enough?
Promiscuity (sleeping around)	Insecurity; anxiety; curiosity; confusion about the part sex plays in forming relationships	Staying out very late or all night; contraceptive devices hidden or obvious taking of the Pill; secrecy concerning a close relationship; rebelliousness	Try to talk about it calmly; be supportive, never react with horror; discuss responsibility and contraception; if you know you can't discuss without embarrassment find someone who can—a friend, your doctor or counsellor
Excessive slimming (affects girls more than boys)	Possible psychological rejection of female sexuality or fear of male sexuality	Bad self-image; consistent loss of weight; starvation due to dislike and refusal of food; self-induced vomiting after being persuaded to eat	Consult doctor/psychologist; be reassuring; don't panic!
Alcohol and drug abuse	Depression; parents do same; too-easy access; defiance of parents; bravado; insecurity; boredom; like the taste; like its effect; identification with drug cultural life-style; denial of, or escape from, real life	*Alcohol:* drunken behaviour *Cannabis:* cough, sore eyes, lethargy *Stimulants:* over-activity, fast, incoherent speech *Hard drugs:* needle marks in arms, scratching due to itching skin, yawning, sweating *Glue:* sores around mouth and nose, drunken behaviour	Check with school; consult doctor/psychologist/counsellor
Rowdiness and vandalism	Proving independence; rejection of home rules in favour of gang's rules; rejection of society's values; rejection of environment	Aggression; acts of violence against property and individuals	Consult psychologist/counsellor

Adrenal glands

Most people have heard of the adrenal glands, but few would claim to know where they are and what they do. They are, in fact, vital to many of the body's normal functions–and are particularly necessary to us in resisting infection and coping with stress.

Q My father suffers from high blood pressure when he gets excited and he is always saying it is the fault of his adrenals. Could this be true?

A Raised blood pressure is one of the symptoms of certain rare adrenal diseases, but such a disease is unlikely to be the cause of your father's problem. Other factors, among them heavy smoking, being overweight or under stress, are much more likely to be responsible for high blood pressure.

If your father is under constant pressure at work, or if he has an excitable temperament, it could be that his adrenals are continually being required to produce adrenalin–the hormone that enables us to cope in emergencies–and consequently his body is not being allowed to return to normal, so the excessive adrenalin in his system could, in time, have led to high blood pressure. But this is not the same as saying that it is the fault of the adrenals themselves.

Q I have been advised to have my adrenals removed. Is it possible to have this done and still live normally?

A Yes. Patients who must have their adrenals removed for medical reasons are able to lead a perfectly normal life by taking cortisone regularly. So you can stop worrying.

Q I have been overweight since I was a child. I have tried dieting, exercise— everything. Could there be something wrong with my adrenal glands that causes this problem?

A If your excess weight is distributed evenly all over your body, the answer must be no. There is only one disease of the adrenals which gives rise to obesity: Cushing's syndrome— and this is extremely rare. It is very easy to spot because there is an obviously uneven distribution of fat on the body: the arms and legs remain thin and fat is concentrated on the chest and abdomen. If you really want to get to the root of your obesity, the first thing you must do is to go and see your doctor.

The adrenal glands–known as the adrenals–are located immediately above the kidneys where they sit, like caps, one on top of each kidney. Each gland consists of two distinct parts: the inner medulla and the outer covering, called the cortex. These parts secrete different hormones, each of which has an entirely separate function.

The adrenal medulla

The medulla, or core of the adrenals is the part of the gland which secretes adrenalin and its close relation, noradrenalin. Together these are known as the 'fight or flight' hormones because they prepare the body for the extra effort required to meet danger, cope with stress or carry out a difficult task.

The adrenal medulla is unique among those hormone-producing glands known as the endocrine glands in that it is closely connected to the nervous system. This is exactly as you would expect of the gland responsible for priming the body to be ready for instant action.

The adrenal glands, which are located just above the kidneys, have two distinct parts performing quite different functions.

Today, the dangers and stresses we face are as likely to be psychological as physical, but either way, the body has the same physical reaction. There is a surge in the production of adrenalin which makes the heart beat faster and more strongly. This raises the blood pressure, while at the same time constricting the blood vessels near the surface of the body and in the gut, re-directing the flow of blood towards the heart–the reason we go 'white with fear'. It also turns glycogen stored in the liver and muscles into glucose required for extra energy.

When the danger is over or the stress removed, adrenalin production is reduced and the body returns to normal. However, if the danger or stress is constant, or if we are continually over-excited or under pressure, the body remains primed for action–and in time this can lead to stress-related conditions (e.g. high blood pressure).

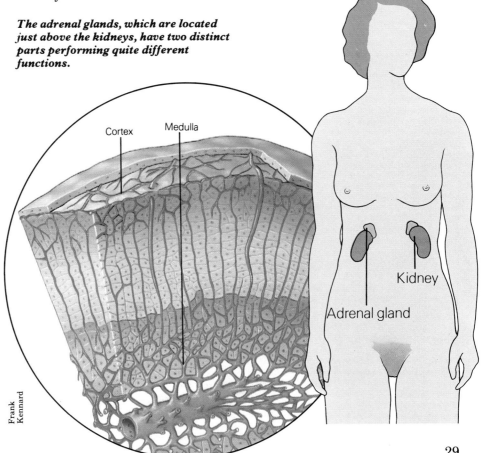

Cortex Medulla

Kidney

Adrenal gland

Frank Kennard

Effects of adrenalin
(the fight or flight hormone) on the body

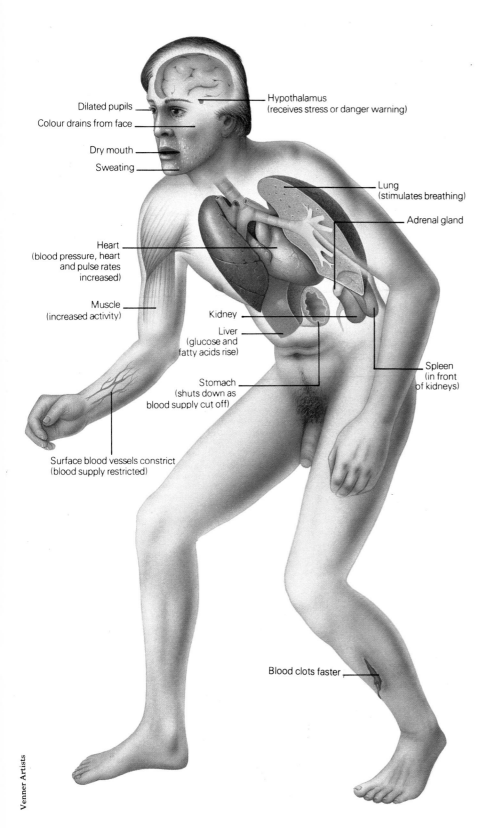

Dilated pupils

Colour drains from face

Dry mouth

Sweating

Hypothalamus
(receives stress or danger warning)

Lung
(stimulates breathing)

Adrenal gland

Heart
(blood pressure, heart
and pulse rates
increased)

Muscle
(increased activity)

Kidney

Liver
(glucose and
fatty acids rise)

Stomach
(shuts down as
blood supply cut off)

Spleen
(in front
of kidneys)

Surface blood vessels constrict
(blood supply restricted)

Blood clots faster

Venner Artists

The adrenal cortex

Wrapped around the adrenal core, the adrenal cortex secretes a series of hormones known as steroids, the most important of which are aldosterone and cortisone.

Aldosterone: There are three types of steroids, each one performing a quite different function. The first, known as the 'salt and water' hormones, increase the water retention in the body. The principal hormone in this category is aldosterone, which acts as a chemical messenger and tells the kidneys to reduce the amount of salt being lost in the urine.

Salt determines the volume of blood in circulation, which in turn affects the heart's efficiency as a pump. Every molecule of salt in the body is accompanied by a large number of water molecules. This means that in losing a lot of salt, the body loses even more water, and this reduces the volume and pressure of the circulating blood. As a result, the heart has difficulty in pumping enough blood around the body.

The secretion of aldosterone is controlled by the hormone renin which is produced by the kidneys. The system works rather like a see-saw: when aldosterone is low, the kidneys produce renin and the hormone level rises; when it is too high, the kidneys reduce their level of activity and the amount of hormone present in the blood returns to a normal level.

Cortisone: The sugar hormones, of which the most important is cortisone, are responsible for raising the level of glucose in the blood. Glucose is the body's principal fuel, and when extra amounts are needed, as in times of stress, cortisone triggers off the conversion of protein into glucose.

Many hormones act to push up the level of sugar in the blood, but cortisone is the most important. By contrast, there is only one hormone that keeps the level down, insulin. Because of this imbalance, there is more likely to be a deficiency, a condition which is known as diabetes and which is treated with insulin in the form of tablets or injections.

As well as playing a key part in metabolism (the life-maintaining processes of the body), cortisone is also vital to the functioning of the immune system, which is the body's defence against illness and injury. But if the normal level of cortisone is raised through medical treatment (for example, to prevent rejection after transplant surgery), the resistance to infection is reduced. However, the body does not produce excessive cortisone naturally.

Sex hormones: The final group of hormones produced by the adrenals are

Hormones and their uses

Source	Hormone	Functions	How synthetic hormones are used as drugs
Adrenal medulla	Adrenalin	Prepares body for physical action (see illustration)	To treat a heart attack In severe allergic collapse During surgery, mixed with local anaesthetic
	Noradrenalin	Maintains even blood pressure	To treat a heart attack
Adrenal cortex	Aldosterone	Regulates excretion of salt by kidney Keeps balance of salt (sodium) and potassium Plays a part in the body's use of carbohydrates	As replacement therapy
	Cortisone	Stimulates manufacture and storage of energy-giving glucose Reduces inflammation Regulates distribution of fat in the body	As replacement therapy when adrenals are missing or defective As replacement therapy when pituitary is defective In shock after severe injuries or burns In severe allergic reactions In rheumatoid arthritis (either as tablets or injected into painful joints) and related diseases In skin diseases such as eczema (as ointment) In anti-cancer treatment, especially when lymphatic system is affected To prevent rejection after transplants
	Sex hormones	Supplement sex hormones secreted by gonads	To correct deficiences In sex-related areas (e.g. contraception) To promote muscle and bone growth

those known as the adrenal sex hormones. These are secreted by the adrenal medulla and they complement those produced in even larger quantities by the gonads, or sex glands.

The principal male sex hormone – also present in women to a lesser degree – is testosterone, which is responsible for increasing the size of muscles. Anabolic steroids are synthetic derivatives of male sex hormones.

This over-excited girl at a pop concert shows many of the physical signs of the effects of adrenalin.

Control of cortisone

Cortisone is so crucial to body function that its secretion needs to be under strict control. The mechanism which regulates its production – and that of steroids – is another endocrine gland, the pituitary, situated at the base of the brain.

The pituitary secretes the hormone ACTH, which stimulates cortisone production and, as with the hormones renin and aldosterone, the two substances work in a see-saw action known as a feedback mechanism. When the cortisone is too low, the pituitary secretes ACTH and the level rises; when it is too high, the gland slows production and the level of cortisone falls.

Cortisone as a drug

Cortisone is used as a replacement treatment in the condition known as Addison's disease, where either the adrenal cortex does not produce sufficient cortisone of its own or the pituitary gland is defective.

As a drug, it is also valuable for a number of other complaints – though it is best used as a short-term remedy. Because it reduces inflammation, it is used in the particularly painful form of arthritis called rheumatoid arthritis and related rheumatoid diseases, for skin complaints such as eczema, and in certain allergic reactions such as asthma or drug allergies.

It is also given to overcome the natural immune reaction so that the body will not reject 'foreign' tissue in transplant operations, and in combination with drugs, to treat cancers.

Steroid therapy is not without its dangers, however. The most serious drawback is that the adrenal cortex is likely to stop producing its own cortisone when synthetic cortisone or a related drug is given for any length of time.

Diseases of the adrenal glands are rare, but occasionally they do go wrong.

Nevertheless, today, with a wide range of replacement hormone treatments serious consequences can be avoided.

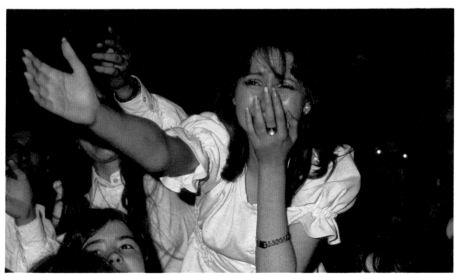

Ageing

Q I am in my twenties and am already a heavy smoker. Will this affect my life expectancy?

A Pulling no punches, the answer has to be yes. Many people underestimate the risk they are taking by smoking 25 cigarettes a day (even low tar brands). Smoking will almost invariably accelerate the ageing process, often causing death before the age of 60 from heart disease and diseases of the lungs and arteries. It is easy to lump together the dangers of car and airplane crashes, stress and obesity, and say that smoking is a minor hazard by comparison. It is not; it is a major cause of premature death.

Q I have always had a very active and satisfactory sex life, and it worries me that I may lose interest as I grow older. Is this likely to happen?

A Not necessarily. Libido does seem to be reduced with old age, but there is no reason for sexual activity to disappear from your life. It is thought that a decrease in sexual desire may be related to the physical changes that occur in the sexual organs with age. After the menopause the vagina is not so well lubricated and a woman may need to use a lubricating jelly to ensure that penetration is easy and painless. An older man will usually find that he is slower to become erect and ejaculate. However, there is no reason for these things to inhibit your lovemaking in later life. Many men and women enjoy sex well into their eighties.

Q I have noticed that my mother who is well into her seventies, has definitely shrunk over the last couple of years. Is this normal?

A Yes. The main reasons for height loss are thinning of the spinal bones and wearing down of the cartilage in between them. Old people's backs also tend to bow slightly, so that they bend forward a little. Trying to maintain a correct posture in earlier life will probably help the vertebrae and the connecting muscles to maintain their strength a little, and this could possibly help to reduce height loss in old age.

The saying 'You're as old as you feel' is more true today than it's ever been because medical advances and improved living conditions are making a healthy and happy old age a reality.

A century ago in Britain a male child who survived his first year could expect to live to be 48, a female 50. Today, many people in the developed world live well into old age. Indeed, the average life expectancy has now reached 70 for men and 76 for women.

Why we live longer

The vast improvement in our life expectancy is largely the result of public health measures. Better sanitation and an improved standard of living have eradicated many of the conditions that tend to encourage disease, and mass immunization programmes have protected children from diseases which killed in the past. New methods of treating disease, such as antibiotics, radiotherapy and transplants, also help save lives.

The increase in the number of older people has led to an expansion in the field of geriatric medicine. Its aim is to alleviate the diseases and disabilities of older people.

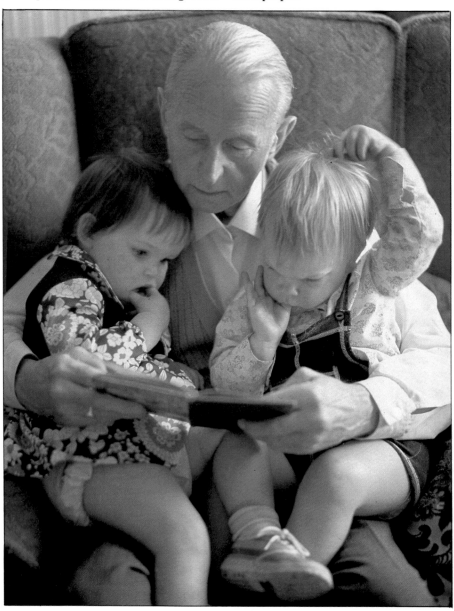

The causes of ageing

The reasons for the differences between people in life expectancy lie in a combination of factors, such as the genes people inherit from their parents (that vital part of cells which determines our inherited characteristics), and their mother's health during pregnancy, both of which can have an effect on longevity. Cigarette smoking and drinking to excess can undermine health, as can living in poor conditions.

Thus the peak of physical, mental, sexual and social well-being varies from person to person and may be greatly influenced by a whole range of elements. For example, a successful businessman may be in his prime at 50, enjoying good health, but if he is made redundant his situation may change overnight – and the psychological effects of being out of work can be far-reaching, causing him to age faster than previously.

The importance of heredity

A person who comes from a long-lived family will generally have a long life, despite any adverse conditions. And just as genetic inheritance has a part to play in determining life expectancy, so, too, it affects the health and strength of individual organs. A 'good' inheritance will mean that a person is more likely to have a strong heart, a healthy brain and sharp eyesight and hearing.

Unfortunately, there is nothing anyone can do about the genes they inherit – no one can choose their parents or go back in time and change them. However, individuals who have inherited 'bad' genes might be able to live out their potential life-span to its full – and live a reasonably long life – if they take care to try and minimize any of the risk factors that cause, or at least contribute to, ill-health and ageing.

Environment

Fortunately, genetic inheritance can only explain some of the traits that appear to run in families. Many physical and mental patterns can only be explained by the shared environment of parents and children. Overweight mothers are more likely to have fat children – though this is more than likely due to their 'inheriting' their mother's eating habits, rather than her genes.

Similarly, bronchitics may have chesty children who grow into bronchitic adults because their parents smoked and there was enough smoke in the home environment to affect the children's lungs. It is also true that they are more likely to imitate their parents and smoke themselves, becoming more liable to lung complaints.

The facts about ageing

- Skin loses its bloom and elasticity, causing wrinkling especially around the eyes and mouth.

- Hair turns grey, then white, becoming sparse – baldness in men starts between 20 and 30, and this is a progressive condition.

- Eyesight deteriorates and eyes are more prone to cataracts.

- A loss of calcium makes bones brittle and liable to fracture. Spinal bones become thinner, resulting in height loss and stooping.

- Loss of teeth, frequently caused through gum disease, alters facial structure.

- The body's balance and gait alters with diminished height and stiffening joints, making the body's carriage less stable.

- Smoking causes heart, circulatory and lung problems.

- Alcohol can damage the liver and nervous system.

And how to stay healthy

- Avoid exposure to the sun and wind. Moisturize and handle the skin gently.

- Keep off certain drugs, like cannabis, in youth – research suggests that this could cause premature hair loss.

- A relatively straightforward operation can cure cataracts.

- Modern advances in hormone treatment can't reverse these changes, but can help to halt or, at least, slow the process down Your doctor will advise you about any risks involved.

- Have regular dental check-ups and maintain an effective oral hygiene routine.

- Take gentle exercise regularly from youth to middle age, older people should avoid strenuous sports – such exertions can cause bones to crack.

- Stop smoking.

- Drink moderately.

The risk of a short life – whether due to inherited or environmental factors – can be greatly reduced if people ensure that they lead a healthy life, especially in later years; eating the right balance of different foods, taking regular exercise, practising routine safety precautions both at home and at work and cutting out smoking can all help to increase potential life-span.

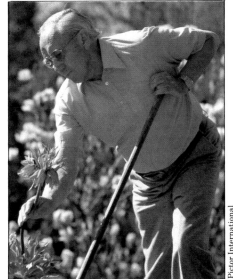

Pictor International

Cell ageing

Common health problems which may increase with age are not in fact caused by the ageing process itself – arthritis has the same causes no matter what the age of the individual. But certain conditions are more likely to occur in later years simply because of a general decline in the body's strength and resistance to infection. This happens as a result of cell ageing.

Most of the body's cells are continually renewing themselves as they wear out. Exact replicas of the old cells are made by a process of cell division, in which cells simply divide into two. The chief exception to this rule is the brain, the cells of which cease division after birth.

As the body ages, the cells begin to deteriorate and function less efficiently, some of which can be explained by general wear and tear on the body. For example, the skin can be compared to a piece of elastic which, on being stretched, will return to its original shape; gradually, with use, it loses its elasticity and remains permanently stretched.

Various theories have been put forward to explain the loss of the body's cellular efficiency. One is that some of the body's cells have a built-in life cycle. A 'programme' switches them on and off – and an example of this can be seen in

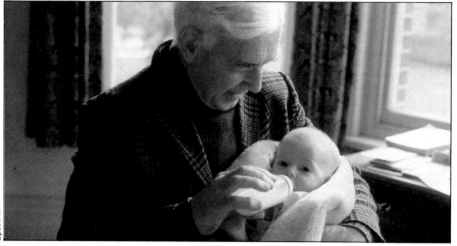

It is important that older people who may otherwise feel isolated experience a continuing sense of involvement and have directions in which to channel their affection. A grandchild, or even a pet, can fulfil that need.

Spectrum

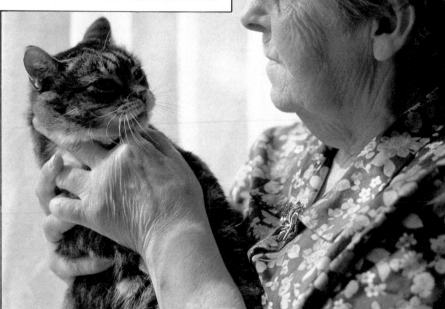

declining muscle strength. In old age certain cells do switch off, causing muscle fibres to decrease in size, but recent research suggests that this decrease can be counteracted, to some extent, by regular exercising throughout middle age and even in later life.

Another theory is called the 'Hayflick limit'. This says that our cells seem to have a predetermined number of cell divisions; once they have divided a certain number of times, they simply stop dividing. Even a small difference in the interval between cell divisions could radically alter a person's life expectancy.

A third theory states that cells gradually fail to reproduce themselves as accurately as before. This can lead to the death of the cell or the production of a whole series of cells which are not as efficient as the original.

The only explanation for the deterioration of brain cells, which are unable to reproduce themselves, is that they just fail to work as efficiently with time, or perhaps as a result of viral diseases.

There is also evidence to suggest that the body's immune system can break down in old age. Normally it produces antibodies which attack foreign cells, which may invade the body as a result of infection, but sometimes the body fails to distinguish foreign cells and it reacts by attacking some of its own cells.

Why women live longer

Women outlive men by an average of five to six years. Various explanations have been given for this, but many of them have little supporting evidence. Some people believe that women are under less stress than men because women usually do not hold such demanding or responsible positions.

Others say that this is nonsense and that quite the reverse is true: women have to deal with far more stress than

men, but they learn to cope with it better.

The fact that, until recently, women have smoked far less than men, could certainly be a contributory factor to female longevity. However, younger women are smoking far more today and this could cause a radical change in their life expectancy.

It has been suggested that female hormones may play a significant part in women's longer life expectancy by protecting them in some way. But research in this area is still inconclusive. However, contrary to this view, there is evidence that the drop in the level of female sex hormones after the menopause can have the opposite effect. The lack of the hormone oestrogen can accelerate wrinkling and cause the vagina to become less well lubricated. Also, the body's calcium balance can be affected and this makes women more susceptible to osteoporosis (thinning of the bones). This condition makes bones

more likely to fracture and can cause bowing of the spine. Hormone replacement therapy can be preventive – although this treatment has some risks which should be carefully considered in consultation with a doctor.

Benefits of retirement

In the past, old people occupied an authoritative and well respected role in society. This role has gradually been undermined, young people being considered more capable of dealing with newer, more scientific methods of working, as well as being thought more creative. One of the effects of these views has been the increase in early retirement – and this can make older people feel useless and unwanted. But in fact many of them find that it gives them the opportunity they have been waiting for to take up new interests and hobbies. The adage 'You're only as old as you feel' may be a cliché, but it rings very true for many people.

AIDS

Q Do you have to be gay to contract AIDS.

A No. Although somewhere between 70 and 80 per cent of sufferers are homosexual, there are three other major groups of people who are likely to get the disease. The first is made up of natives of Haiti, where the disease seems to have taken hold in the general population; about five per cent of cases in the United States occur in Haitians. The second major group at risk are drug addicts, who form about 17 per cent of known cases. The third group consists of haemophiliacs. Isolated cases of infection from blood transfusions have been reported.

Q Is it possible for children to get AIDS?

A Unfortunately yes. The largest group of children identified to date have come from Miami. Of the nine Miami children found to have AIDS, most were children of mothers who came from Haiti. Only one of the mothers definately had AIDS but blood tests from others suggested that they might have problems similar to AIDS. In children, the disease occurs in infancy and is presumably passed from the mother to the foetus during pregnancy. These are nearly always children of drug addicts, or of mothers who have had sexual relationships with bisexual men.

Q I quite often go to the United States on business or holiday trips. I am gay and lead an active sex life, what is the chance of catching AIDS?

A If you are involved in any type of homosexual activity while you are there, then you are definitely at risk.

Q Is AIDS inevitably fatal, or is there a less serious form?

A A death rate for patients in whom AIDS is established is probably around 70 per cent. However it is possible that many people have AIDS in a less serious form, and that the conditions we now call AIDS is only the most serious form of the disease.

When a new killer disease suddenly starts to attack more and more people, the resources of medical science rise to the challenge. So far, progress towards a cure has been slow but more is being learnt all the time.

Few events in recent medical history have been so dramatic or caused so much confusion as the emergence of the disease popularly known as AIDS. This disease was first recognized in 1981, although it had appeared in the United States two years earlier. Since then it has occurred in Europe and has reached epidemic proportions in certain parts of the American community. So far, there are no signs that either a cure or way of preventing it have been found. However, in the few years since its recognition doctors and scientists have discovered a great deal about the course of the disease and the people who at present appear to be at risk of developing it.

What is AIDS?

AIDS – Acquired Immune Deficiency Syndrome – is a new type of immunodeficiency disease. An immunodeficiency disease is one that affects the functioning of the body's immune defence system. The body depends on this system to ward off organisms, such as bacteria or viruses, that cause infection. Under normal circumstances it identifies disease-carrying organisms as abnormal and then activates the release of substances called antibodies to attack and destroy them.

It appears that AIDS affects the body's ability to destroy some types of organisms in its cells. This results in the development of certain unusual forms of infection. These are known as opportunistic infections — infections that result from organisms whose ability to cause a disease is increased when the body's resistance is lowered. An opportunistic infection that is quite common is a type of pneumonia caused by the organism *Pneumocystis carinii*. Pneumocystis carinii pneumonia (PCP) previously occured only rarely.

AIDS can also result in the development of rare tumours, notably Kaposi's sarcoma. This usually affects the skin only but in AIDS patients may spread throughout the body. Although the reason for the presence of Kaposi's sarcoma in AIDS is unknown, some authorities believe that it is probably also due to a deficiency in the immune system. The development of Kaposi's sarcoma and one of the opportunistic infections such as PCP are two main features of AIDS. Although other rare tumours may be found, patients nearly always have either Kaposi's sarcoma or an opportunistic infection, or both.

During Gay Pride Week in New York in 1983, homosexuals took to the streets in an attempt to get the authorities to pour more money into research on AIDS. So far, no effective form of treatment exists to combat this killer disease.

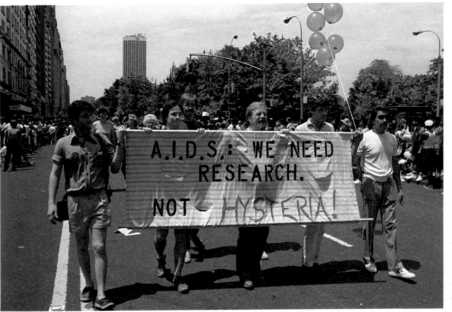

One of the most disturbing aspects of AIDS is that it occurs in people with no known history of immunodeficiency and is therefore an acquired, rather than a congenital (present at birth) disease; in many cases AIDS affects young people who previously appeared to be healthy.

The victims

The majority of people who suffer from AIDS are male homosexuals. In the United States about 70 per cent of AIDS victims fall into this category. Drug addicts who inject themselves with drugs make up about another 17 per cent. Curiously, natives of Haiti are also prone to the disease, although it is mainly Haitian men who are infected – about six per cent of all known cases in the United States are Haitians.

Small numbers of other people are also known to be at risk, notably heterosexual partners of bisexual men and intravenous drug abusers, as well as haemophiliacs and other people who need treatment with blood products.

The effect of AIDS seems to vary between the various groups at risk. For example, 50 per cent of affected homosexual men get Kaposi's sarcoma, but only about 10 per cent of the patients from other groups exhibit this cancer.

How common is AIDS?

The unusual combination of Kaposi's sarcoma and PCP was first noticed simultaneously in Los Angeles and New York. Once it was established that this combination resulted from a new disease

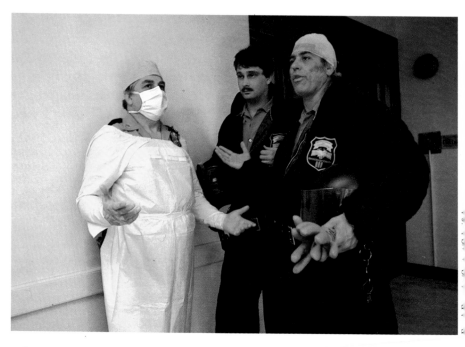

it became clear that a few cases had existed as early as 1979.

From such small beginnings the disease has spread at an alarming rate, and in the United States approximately 50 new cases are reported to the Centres for Disease Control weekly. By the end of 1983 almost 3000 cases had been reported and the number is doubling every six months. This means that by the summer of 1984 there will be about 6000 cases.

In Europe AIDS is much less common. In October 1983 the World Health Organization reported 267 European cases.

At Westchester County Medical Centre in Valhalla, New York, staff who deal with AIDS victims have demanded specially made protective clothing.

Causes

When AIDS was thought to be a disease exclusively affecting male homosexuals, it was suggested that the frequent attacks of venereal disease to which many homosexuals are prone 'wore out' the immune system and made it ineffectual. A second theory for its cause was the widespread use among male homo-

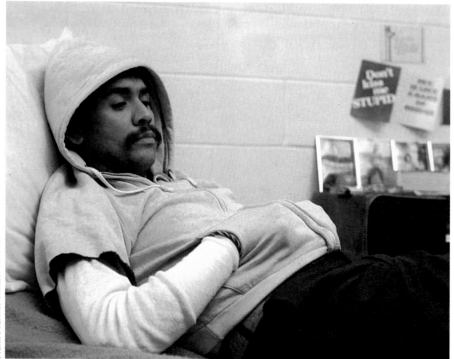

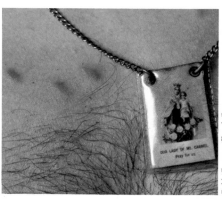

Kaposi's Sarcoma (above) is a rare form of cancer, and before the emergence of AIDS, it was rarely found in young men. Homosexual men are more prone to this particular sign of AIDS.

The young AIDS' victim (left) contracted the disease through the use of intra-venous drugs. Drug users also run a high risk of contacting hepatitis B – both these conditions occur when dirty needles are used to inject drugs.

sexuals of a group of drugs of abuse known as nitrates. However, as the number of heterosexual patients increased both of these theories were largely abandoned.

One of the most interesting aspects of the disease is that, with the exception of Haitian men, the same groups of people who are at risk of contracting it are also at special risk of contracting Hepatitis B. Hepatitis B can be spread by blood transfusion and also by the use of dirty needles such as hypodermic or tattooing needles. It also appears to enter the bloodstream during sexual intercourse.

Hepatitis B is caused by a virus, and the similarity between groups at risk from it and AIDS has suggested that a virus may also be responsible for AIDS. If this theory is correct, it is possible that the virus would be passed on during sexual activity or, in the case of drug addicts and haemophiliacs, by direct injection of infected blood.

Recent studies suggest a causative role for HTLV (Human T-cell Leukemia Virus) and a French group has discovered increased incidences of infection by an agent which they call "Lymphadeno-pathy-associated virus". These two agents may prove to be the same or closely related.

Little is known about the incubation period of AIDS; it may be very long – probably a matter of one to four years. And it is not known whether everyone who becomes infected actually fully develops the syndrome.

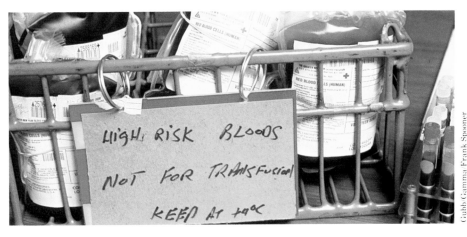

Since it was discovered that AIDS could be transmitted through blood transfusion, great efforts have been made to discourage high-risk donors from giving blood.

Symptoms

AIDS usually begins with a long period of ill health, but in each case the symptoms of AIDS are those that are typical of the opportunistic infections or the development of a rare tumour. For example, weight loss and diarrhoea are symptoms of opportunistic infections that affect the intestines, and coughing and shortness of breath occur with PCP infection.

While a great variety of other infections may then develop, the common ones appear to be infestation of the mouth and oesophagus with Candida – the fungal organism that causes thrush – and cyto-megalo virus infection, which, when present alone, usually gives rise to an illness similar to glandular fever.

Treatment and prevention

At the moment, there is very little that doctors can do to halt the process of AIDS – treatment consists of trying to meet the infections as they occur with antibiotics which may be effective against the organisms that cause them. In the case of prevention, given that the disease is caused by a virus, the ideal approach would be to find the virus concerned and make a vaccine that would give immunity to it. Some groups are studying the use of Interferon to repair damage to the immune system.

With no effective cure available, it is particularly important that AIDS victims are given careful counselling to help them come to terms with their condition.

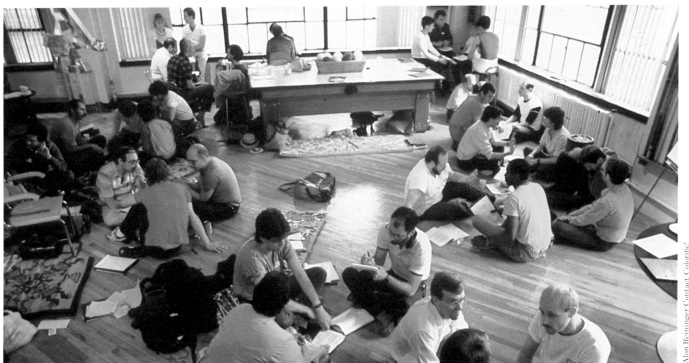

Alcoholism

Q I have heard that women are more at risk when they drink than men. Is there any truth in this?

A Drinking among women is on the increase. Not only is it now accepted that they can go into bars on their own, but they can also buy alcohol from the supermarket. Generally speaking, however, women still drink less than men—and so they come to less harm. But if a woman becomes an alcoholic she is more vulnerable to the effects than a man; her liver is likely to be affected earlier than a man's, and treatment is often not as satisfactory. Then there is the problem of the alcoholic expectant mother—she risks causing mental retardation in her baby, and it may also be born with congenital deformities such as dislocation of the hips or a cleft palate.

Q My brother-in-law drinks an awful lot, and in the last year I have noticed a marked change in his personality. He used to be pleasant and outgoing—now he is surly and introverted. Could his drinking be the cause of this?

A Almost certainly. Very heavy drinkers can become moody, violent and jealous, or think they are being persecuted. Even worse, they can have trouble in remembering things, they may hear imaginary voices, see visions and become unable to cope with life. All this can result in *delirium tremens*, the symptoms of which are trembling, sweating and a feeling of panic. If you recognize any of these danger signs in your brother-in-law, he should be encouraged to seek help as soon as possible.

Q Where can I go to get help for alcoholism?

A Go to your doctor for advice on the physical aspects of alcohol addiction—he or she will refer you to a clinic if necessary. For family problems—and any others you may have—see a social worker. There are also self-help groups such as Alcoholics Anonymous, who can provide long-term help and support for anyone who wants to kick the habit.

Most people drink moderately, enjoy it, and come to no harm. But there are those who become so dependent on alcohol that they are unable to lead a normal life. This makes it vital to recognize the danger signals and to know when to stop.

When people talk about alcohol, they are usually referring to drinks which contain varying amounts of pure alcohol. Alcoholic drinks have a restricted food value in the form of sugar (as in sweet wines, for example) and carbohydrate (in spirits and beers made from grain), but basically alcohol is a drug—that is, a substance which affects the workings of the mind and body.

Taken in moderation, alcohol can encourage the appetite and produce a feeling of well-being. This is because the alcohol stimulates the blood flow to the skin which has the effect of making the drinker feel pleasantly warm. When it reaches the brain anxiety is reduced and self-confidence increases.

Dependency

Heavy drinking, however, is quite another matter. If it is repeated over any period of time, subtle changes can occur in the personality—it is thought that these have a chemical basis—and this can lead to the need to carry on the drinking pattern. When this feeling becomes so persistent that every time a drink is delayed there is an urgent desire to have another, a state known as 'dependency' has been reached.

In the early stages of heavy drinking, this dependency tends to be psychological rather than physical. After all, it is anxiety and stress that usually lead people into drinking in the first place, but then they come to rely on the alcohol as a

Drinking in relation to age and sex

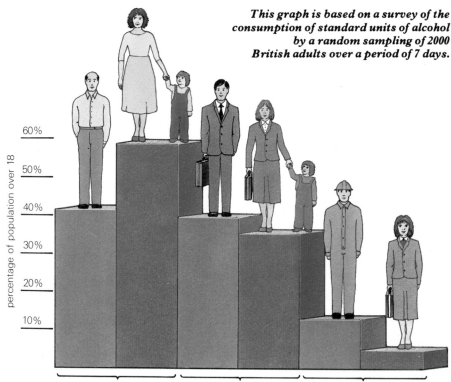

This graph is based on a survey of the consumption of standard units of alcohol by a random sampling of 2000 British adults over a period of 7 days.

percentage of population over 18

60%
50%
40%
30%
20%
10%

light drinking
men 1-10 units
women 1-5

moderate
men 11-50 units
women 6-35

heavy drinking
over 50 units for men
over 35 units for women

prop to keep them at their ease.

Unfortunately, if the drinking becomes increasingly heavier, psychological dependence can give way to a physical dependence. In the transitional period this may not be noticeable, but as physical dependence grows, withdrawal will become more and more difficult and uncomfortable. Eventually, deprivation for any length of time will result in trembling, sweating and acute stress. The first drink will always relieve these feelings—until the next time.

Alcohol and personality changes

Alcohol tends to affect different people in different ways. The same amount can turn one person into the 'life and soul' of the party, bring out violent aggression in another, and merely send a third quietly to sleep.

Although it reduces tension, alcohol is not a stimulant, but a depressant. As soon as it enters the bloodstream, it begins to impair judgement, self-control and skill. Research has shown that workers with blood alcohol levels of between 30mg (the equivalent of one pint of beer) and 100mg have considerably more accidents than those with less than 30mg.

With driving, the likelihood of having an accident increases when the blood alcohol level reaches 30mg; at 80mg, it is four times greater; and at 150mg (about five pints of beer) it is 25 times greater. This is because the co-ordination between hand and eye and the ability to judge distances deteriorates progressively.

The problems of alcoholism

Once an excessive drinker is unable to stop drinking without outside help, he or she can be classified as an alcoholic. And it is in this situation that the social, economic and medical problems—often already self-evident in the heavy drinker—can worsen, bringing despair and confusion to the life of the alcoholic—and everyone else with whom he or she has contact.

Alcohol breaks up marriages, sets children against parents, and vice-versa, and costs individuals their jobs and their reputation in the community. Ultimately, of course, it can also kill.

When most people think of alcoholics, they visualize meths drinkers and down-and-out inebriates, but it is not just the deprived and inadequate members of our society that resort to the bottle as a means of escape—there are children too inebriated to take in their school lessons after lunch, businessmen incapable of working in the afternoons, and house-wives barely able to prepare a meal at the end of the day.

Alcoholism can strike irrespective of age, class, creed, colour or sex, and once afflicted, alcoholics will mix only with like-minded friends, neglect their families, break promises, lie and steal, and live only to drink.

Reasons for heavy drinking

Drinking is an accepted and approved cultural activity. As such, it would appear that some people are more exposed to the risk of becoming alcoholics than others simply because of social pressures and conditioning. For example, studies of national groups reveal that the Irish have a high rate of alcoholism; in contrast, the Jews' is very low. Certain professions seem to encourage alcoholism—travelling salesmen, barpeople and company directors, among others, are particularly at risk. Presumably, extensive socializing and the availability of drink are responsible in these cases.

The housewife is increasingly a victim of this form of addiction. Often isolated, either with small children or with too little to do once a family has grown up and left home, drinking can provide her with a welcome escape from an apparently humdrum existence. And the fact that most supermarkets today stock alcohol makes it only too easy for her to buy it as part of her routine shopping.

In most cases, drinking starts at an early age, with children, not surprisingly, copying the habits of their parents. It is

A single whisky and a glass of wine each represent a standard unit of alcohol. Most people are unaware that a pint of beer is equal to twice this amount.

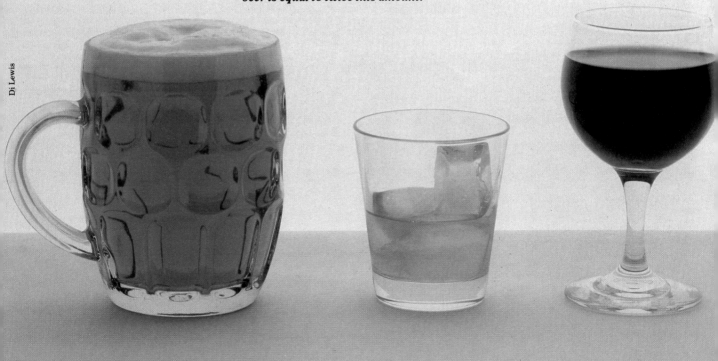

Di Lewis

The effects of alcoholism

Physical

● Cirrhosis of the liver—there is no cure for this most common disease associated with alcoholism
● Other diseases—alcoholics commonly develop peptic ulcers, kidney trouble and heart disease
● Pins and needles in hands and feet
● Loss of appetite and insomnia make individual weak and tired
● Attacks of trembling and sweating when alcohol is withdrawn
● Delirium tremens—more serious form of attack after withdrawal, accompanied by frightening hallucinations

Emotional and Social

● Alcoholics suffer increasingly from anxiety, depression, remorse and phobic fears
● Obsession with drink overrides all else of importance in life and the need for drink increases as tolerance grows
● Disruption or breakdown of family life. Loss of friends and interests
● Lack of concentration and loss of memory
● Loss of efficiency and reliability at work may lead to possible job loss
● Neglect of personal appearance. Chronic alcoholics seek the company of others like themselves

statistically proven that the children of alcoholic parents have a higher than average risk of developing the problem themselves. Teenagers also tend to be strongly influenced by their friends' behaviour.

Today, so much socializing is built around the consumption of alcohol that it is hard to avoid it. You may easily find yourself mixing with others who drink, going to the same place regularly for this purpose, becoming accustomed to the sights, sounds and smells. In addition, advertising suggests that men are not men unless they drink, and drunkenness is a sign of masculinity. Finally, a refusal to drink is usually considered to be abnormal and often seen as a deliberately anti-social action. All these factors can

Drinking with friends is a relaxing way to unwind. However, when drinking is done for its own sake, or people are reluctant to stop no matter how much they've drunk — it's time they stopped to consider the risks to health, family, work and social life.

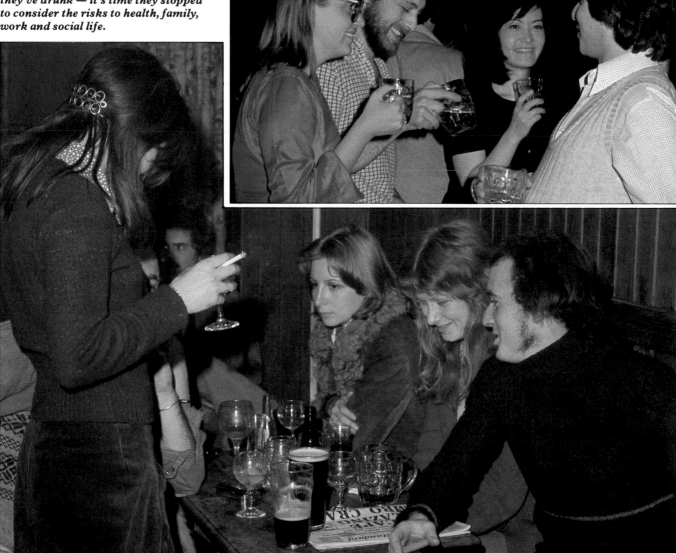

A **What is the best cure for a hangover? I get a terrible headache and everyone has different ideas on what I should do about it.**

A The only real cure for a hangover is rest. Paracetamol may be used to treat a bad headache, but aspirin should be left well alone. It will only cause further disturbance to an already irritated stomach. The 'hair of the dog' remedy (having another drink) is not recommended: it will simply lead to spending the rest of the day in bed in a drunken haze. As you say, everyone has their own pet cure—orange juice, vitamin pills, egg in milk etc., but the rule to follow is that prevention is better than cure. Drink as much water as possible before going to sleep after a drinking session. Dehydration is the main cause of a hangover and water will help reduce this effect of alcohol. But (to pursue the subject to its obvious conclusion) it is still best to try not to drink too much and to avoid having hangovers altogether.

Q **Are some people more vulnerable to alcohol than others? I seem to get drunk on one glass of wine.**

A It used to be thought that people who found themselves in trouble over drinking were different in their physical and psychological makeup to others, but this is now thought to be untrue. Anyone can become an alcoholic and if you find you do not respond too well to alcohol, try to avoid it. If everyone knew their limits and stuck to them firmly, the problem of alcoholism with all its risks would be greatly reduced.

Q **My sister says her husband has a drinking problem, but denies that he is an alcoholic. Is this possible?**

A No. They are one and the same thing. Someone whose drinking over a period of time has made him dependent on drink and who may do harm to himself and others is an alcoholic—though he and his family may not wish to see the real nature of the condition. But sooner or later—and the sooner the better—they are going to have to face it for what it is.

combine to make it difficult to maintain a responsible attitude to alcohol.

Danger signals
The body develops a tolerance to alcohol, and the danger lies in the fact that more drinks are soon needed to reproduce the original feeling of relaxation and well-being. The higher the daily intake becomes, the more difficult it is to give it up. If an individual drinks to relieve worries, this can lead to an escalation in drinking: more worries mean more alcohol, and fewer worries become the reason for a round of celebratory drinks.

It can take between 10 and 15 years for someone to develop an addiction to the point where they can be classified as an alcoholic. But symptoms to watch for are an obvious obsession with alcohol and the inability to give it up or even restrict drinking to a reasonable level, moral and physical deterioration, and obvious work, money and family problems. The typical alcoholic will probably need a drink early in the morning and may need continual boosters to keep going during the day.

Safe drinking
In a situation where an individual wants to drink, but not to excess, alcohol should be consumed as slowly as possible and some food should always be eaten beforehand so that the alcohol will be absorbed more slowly into the blood-stream. Consumption can also be kept down by interspersing alcoholic drinks with non-alcoholic ones. It is better not to drink alone, as it is all too easy to consume more than usual just in order to combat feelings of loneliness.

If you do not want to drink, you should not feel shy about saying no. And if you know how much you can drink before going over the top, simply set a limit to the number of drinks you accept and stick to it.

Finally, the combination of drinking and driving—or handling any type of machinery—is known to be lethal and is recognized as such by law. Those who have more than two-and-a-half pints or doubles prior to driving make themselves liable to prosecution; paradoxically, if this amount is consumed slowly, throughout the day, no harm will be done. This is because the body is able to eliminate the alcohol, in advance of any build up in the bloodstream.

People who know that they are going to drink should not travel by car; or, alternatively, they should take someone with them who does not drink to drive them home. Otherwise it is sensible for them to leave the car where it is and get a lift or take a cab. There are no half measures in this instance; the rule is clear and simple: *never drink and drive.*

What is harmful drinking?

Regular drinkers can easily progress from one drinking stage to the next — so they should know what amount is harmful.

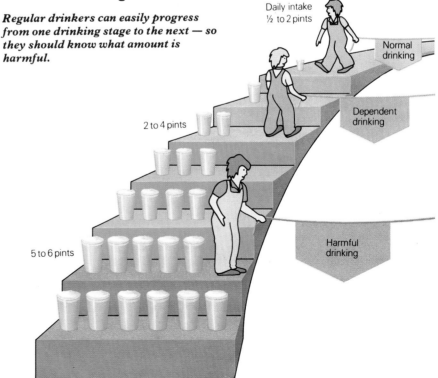

Venner Artists

Alimentary canal

Q My baby always seems to get hiccups after a feed. Why is this?

A This is nothing that you need worry about. Hiccups are perfectly normal in a well-fed baby. They are caused by a lack of synchronization between the up and down movements of the muscle sheets at the base of the chest (the diaphragm) and those of the flap called the epiglottis which shuts off the airway during swallowing. An over-full stomach seems to be one cause of hiccups, so try giving smaller feeds more often.

Q My grandmother always insisted on our chewing our food 20 times before we were allowed to swallow it. Why did she do this?

A Basically, chewing food well—though perhaps not 20 times—aids digestion. It makes food moist and easier to swallow. It is also particularly important for the digestion of fruits and vegetables because the nutrients in these foods are wrapped in a substance called cellulose which is impossible for humans to digest. The grinding action of the teeth during chewing unlocks these nutrients. Once it gets into the stomach and intestines, food is broken down by a whole range of chemicals which cannot get right to the heart of big chunks of food. This is another reason why thorough chewing helps the alimentary canal do its job.

Q Sometimes my new baby is sick so violently that vomit shoots right across the room. Is this normal?

A No. This sounds like projectile vomiting, as doctors call it. You should see your doctor straightaway as it could be serious. Projectile vomiting in babies of two to three weeks old is very often a sign of a disorder called pyloric stenosis, a thickening of the channel at the far end of the stomach, where it leads into the small intestine. This thickening means that food cannot easily get out of the stomach and is therefore forcibly ejected. But a simple operation can usually put the problem right.

The alimentary canal is where our food is digested. We are mainly unaware of this important process—so what exactly happens?

Food is the fuel that powers the activities of the body. But before it can be of any use, it must be properly processed. The body's food processing plant is the alimentary canal, a muscular tube about 10m (33 ft) long which starts at the mouth and ends at the anus, from which undigested wastes are expelled in the form of faeces.

Eating

When food is put in the mouth at the beginning of its journey through the alimentary canal, it is tested for taste and temperature by the tongue. Solid food is bitten off by the front teeth (incisors), then chewed by the back teeth or molars. Even before the food is tasted, and during chewing, saliva pours into the mouth from salivary glands near the lower jaw.

Saliva moistens food, and the enzymes it contains start digestion. By the time it is ready to be swallowed, the original mouthful has been transformed into a soft ball, called a bolus, and warmed or cooled to the right temperature.

Though quick, this stage is in fact quite complex. First the tongue pushes the bolus of food up against the roof of the mouth and into the muscle-lined cavity at the back of the mouth: the pharynx.

Once food is in the pharynx, several activities take place within the space of a couple of seconds to prevent swallowing from interfering with breathing. The soft palate, the non-bony part of the roof of the mouth, is pushed upwards by the tongue to shut off the inner entrance to the nose, the vocal cords are quickly drawn together, and a flap of tissue called the epiglottis snaps down over the entrance to the tubes that lead to the lungs.

From the pharynx the bolus now passes into the oesophagus, or gullet, the tube joining the mouth to the stomach. The bolus does not just fall down the oesophagus because of gravity but is pushed along by waves of muscle action called peristalsis.

Except during eating, the oesophagus is kept closed just above where it enters the stomach by a ring of muscle called the cardiac sphincter which prevents the highly acid contents of the stomach from being regurgitated into the oesophagus. As a bolus of food passes down the oesophagus, the sphincter relaxes to open the pathway into the stomach, which relaxes in preparation for being filled.

Peristalsis—how partially digested food (chyme) is moved through the intestine

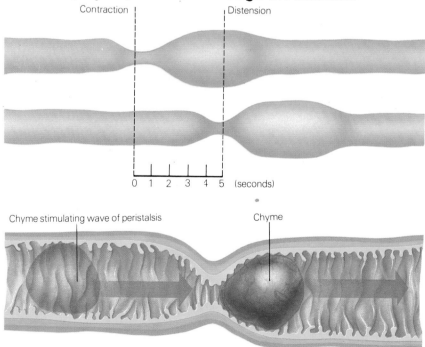

Contraction | Distension

0 1 2 3 4 5 (seconds)

Chyme stimulating wave of peristalsis

Chyme

Alimentary canal

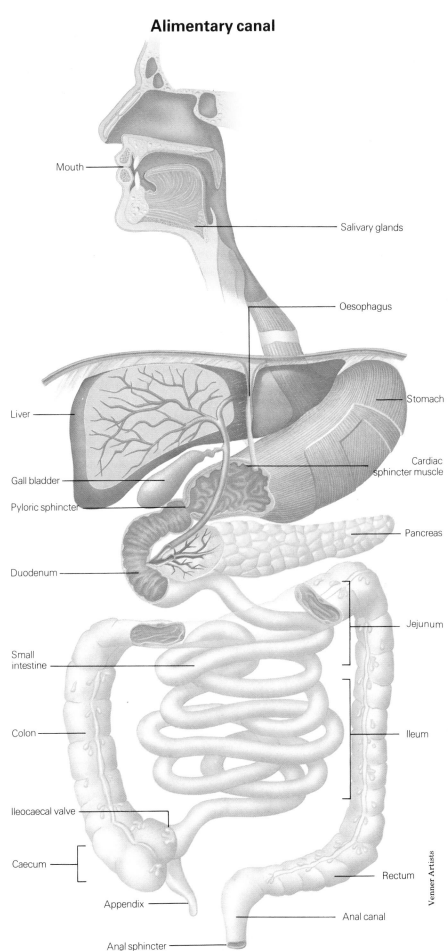

Mouth

Salivary glands

Oesophagus

Liver

Stomach

Cardiac
sphincter muscle

Gall bladder

Pyloric sphincter

Pancreas

Duodenum

Jejunum

Small
intestine

Colon

Ileum

Ileocaecal valve

Caecum

Rectum

Appendix

Anal canal

Anal sphincter

Venner Artists

Digestion

The stomach is a collapsible muscular bag designed to store food (so that it is not usually necessary to eat small meals all day long), to mix food with various digestive juices, then to release it slowly into the intestine.

Food is mixed as the stomach wall contracts and relaxes and is moved along by waves of peristalsis. By the time it has spent two to six hours being processed in the stomach, the partially digested food has been converted by various chemicals to a liquid called chyme.

The stomach exit is guarded by a muscle known as the pyloric sphincter, very like the sphincter at the stomach entrance, except that it is never completely closed. As the waves of peristalsis push chyme through the stomach, the

Aids to digestion

The alimentary canal processes approximately 35 tons of food during the course of an average life of 70 years. No wonder, then, that it sometimes goes wrong. Some ills of the alimentary canal are so common they have become household words—ulcers, appendicitis, constipation, diarrhoea and heartburn, to name a few. While some are unavoidable, there are ways to keep the digestive system healthy.

● Do not eat (or feed children) too much. This puts a strain on the digestion and can create a weight problem. In infants it can lead to vomiting and regurgitation.

● Chew your food properly before swallowing. The digestion of carbohydrates starts in the mouth with ptyalin, an enzyme in saliva.

● Include sufficient roughage in your diet—fruit with the skin on, lightly cooked vegetables, bran with your breakfast cereal. Dietary fibre cannot be digested by the alimentary canal but stimulates the passage of food through the large intestine, helping to prevent constipation and perhaps some intestinal diseases as well. Fibre-rich foods are useful for slimming because they are filling, but not fattening.

● Drink sparingly with meals because liquids of any kind dilute digestive juices.

● Avoid any foods you know you or your family react to badly.

● Minimize stress. This increases the acid secretion of the stomach and the muscular action of the whole system, causing food to be pushed along too fast so that it is not properly digested.

● Stop smoking, or cut down, because, like stress, it stimulates acid secretion.

Common problems in babies and children

Symptom	Related symptoms	Possible causes	Action
Diarrhoea **Babies**	Fever, appetite loss, vomiting	Infection of canal or middle ear, tonsillitis, common cold	Boiled water only, call doctor if symptoms persist more than 24 hours
		Food allergy	Boiled water only. Re-introduce foods one by one to find cause. See doctor it if persists
Diarrhoea **Children**	Fever, appetite loss, vomiting, abdominal pain	Infection of canal	Fluids for 24 hours. See doctor if symptoms persist
		Effects of antibiotic drug	Bland diet; fluids. See doctor if symptoms persist
Vomiting **Babies**	Diarrhoea, appetite loss	Too much air taken in with feed	Teat with smaller hole. Small, frequent feeds
	Constipation	Bowel obstruction	See doctor at once
Projectile vomiting **Babies under two months**	Constipation, no appetite loss	Pyloric stenosis (see questions)	See doctor at once
Vomiting **Children**	Diarrhoea, appetite loss, abdominal pain	Appendicitis	See doctor at once
Constipation **Babies**	Vomiting	Bowel obstruction	See doctor at once
		Anxiety about potty training	Stop training temporarily
Constipation **Children**	Poor appetite	Lack of fluids, lack of exercise, too little roughage	Plenty of fluids; increase roughage

How long food is in the body

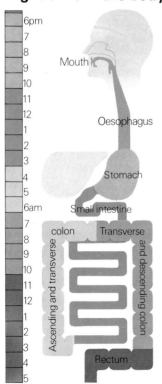

sphincter lets out chyme in small amounts into the small intestine.

The small intestine is in fact the longest section of the alimentary canal, measuring 20ft (6m) and getting its name not from its length but its width—about 1½in (4cm). The first 10in (25cm) of the small intestine is known as the duodenum, the next 8ft (2.5cm) as the jejunum and the final 11ft (3.3m) as the ileum.

The largest part of the digestive process takes place in the small intestine, through the action of digestive juices made not only by the intestine itself, but by the liver and the pancreas which are closely linked to the alimentary canal. The liver produces bile, a substance stored by the gall bladder and needed to digest fats, and the pancreas produces pancreatic secretions, which, like bile, pass into the duodenum.

As waves of peristalsis move chyme along the small intestine, it is given another thorough mixing. In the ileum, digested foodstuffs are absorbed into the blood via thousands of tiny corrugations in the gut wall called villi and carried first to the liver, then to all body cells. At the end of the ileum a sphincter called the ileocaecal valve keeps chyme trapped in the small intestine until another meal is eaten. When more food enters the stomach, the valve opens and chyme passes into the large intestine, a tube about 3ft (1.5m) long and an average 7.5 cm (3 in) in diameter.

Excretion

Anatomists divide the large intestine into four parts: the caecum, colon, rectum and anal canal. The caecum, and the worm-like appendix that extends from it, are both blind alleys with no known functions in man. In the colon, by far the largest section at 1.3 m (4½ ft), water is absorbed into the blood from the liquid remains of digestion. By the time these remains reach the rectum, they are in the form of solid faeces. Rather than the continuous contractions of peristalsis, the progressively more solid remains are moved along by giant propulsions that take place only a few times a day.

Finally, faeces enter the anal canal, which is kept closed by the last sphincter in the alimentary canal. In infancy the sphincter opens automatically when the anal canal is full. But as the nervous system matures, we learn to override the automatic signals.

Allergies

Q I have been suffering from a food allergy for years and sometimes it really gets on top of me. What I want to know is can there be a lasting cure?

A There are several ways of relieving the symptoms of allergies, but they are not cures. Whatever treatment you receive, it is not going to change your basic sensitivity to the particular food in question.

Q My daughter's best friend has just developed an allergy to penicillin, and has terrified my daughter by claiming that she will die at the onset of the first disease she catches, as she won't be able to take penicillin to fight the infection. Surely there must be some alternative drugs to pencillin?

A There is really no need to worry. Although a penicillin allergy does reduce the number of antibiotics which a doctor might consider prescribing, there is still a range of antibiotics available for those people with this type of allergy.

Q My son of four is allergic to cats and touching them brings him out in a nasty rash. Will he grow out of this problem or will it remain with him for life?

A Possibly. Children who suffer from either allergic rashes or eczema often do grow out of those problems though they may suffer from other forms of allergy (asthma for example) when they are older because they have a basic tendency to be allergic.

Q I suffer terribly from hay fever and, as I am now pregnant, I am anxious to know whether my child could possibly inherit this condition from me?

A Unfortunately, this could happen, although it is by no means a certainty. Research shows that children of allergic parents are more likely to suffer from an allergy than other children. But there are still not enough facts available for us to fully understand why this should be so.

Allergy-sufferers sometimes have to bear considerable discomfort and inconvenience, but although there are at present no cures for allergies, medical research is making encouraging progress in discovering the many causes and alleviating the symptoms

An allergy is a sensitivity to a substance which does not normally cause people any discomfort or harm. Hay fever, which is caused by a sensitivity to pollen, is a well-known example. Asthma, eczema, rashes and a variety of other complaints can be caused partly or entirely by an allergy. In fact, allergies can affect almost any part of the body and be caused by a vast range of natural and artificial substances.

They are seldom life-threatening, though they can be dangerous, and are often very uncomfortable for the sufferer. They are also a great puzzle to medical science, because although many allergic conditions can be relieved by medical treatment, we still have very little idea of their basic cause.

Allergies are a reaction to allergens, a name given to those substances (such as

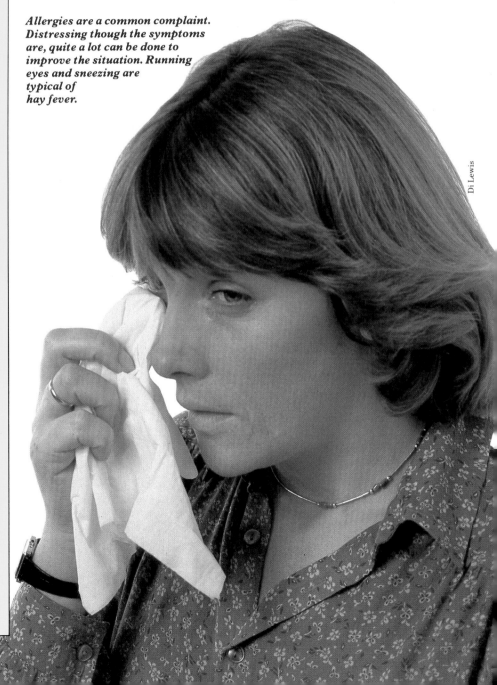

Allergies are a common complaint. Distressing though the symptoms are, quite a lot can be done to improve the situation. Running eyes and sneezing are typical of hay fever.

Di Lewis

pollen) that spark off symptoms of an allergy in someone who is sensitive to it. Among the commonest allergens are foods (notably eggs, milk and fish), pollens, spores, insect bites (especially bee and wasp stings), animal fluff (such as cat's hair) and chemicals. One type of allergy is caused by contact with metals, which explains why some people get a nasty rash from wearing certain pieces of jewellery.

A common allergen in the home is the dust mite, a tiny creature, invisible to the naked eye, which lives in bedclothes, carpets and curtains. Some people are allergic to heat or cold so that their hands swell when plunged, for example, into hot or cold water.

Symptoms

As a general rule, the symptoms of an allergy tend to show up in those parts of the body which are exposed to the allergen. So an airborne allergen, like pollen, makes its severest impact in the eyes, nose and air passages. Food allergies reveal themselves through swollen lips, stomach upsets or diarrhoea.

An allergy to a metal would affect the skin, and an allergy to rubber would result in a rash on part of your body where, for example, the elastic of your underwear came into contact with your skin. But this is only a general rule, because if an allergen gets into the bloodstream it can cause reactions almost anywhere.

This is particularly true of food allergens, which are absorbed through the digestive tract into the blood. Because of this, food allergens can cause a wide range of reactions in sufferers, including eczema, nettlerash, asthma and even mental disorders.

Skin allergies: There are really three basic forms of allergic reaction affecting the skin. The most common, particularly among children, is eczema and this appears as a rash or as scaly skin, to be found mostly on the hands, face, neck and the creases of the forearms and behind the knees.

Contact dermatitis, often caused by metal jewellery or by chemicals in washing powders, is a blistery, itchy inflammation of skin which has come into direct contact with the allergen.

Then there is urticaria, best described by its popular name, nettlerash. This is a red, irritating swelling which often has a small white point in the middle which makes it look like a nettle sting.

Eye and ear allergies: Allergic reactions can also affect the eye, and these generally show up as irritation and redness in the white of the eye. Severe

swellings can occur, but generally the symptoms are watering and soreness.

The ears, too, are sometimes the target of allergens; when this happens fluid will build up inside the ear and may temporarily affect your hearing.

Hayfever can affect the eyes and ears, though its principal target is the nose, which becomes stuffy, runny or sneezy. Unlike a common cold, which should clear up after four or five days in an otherwise healthy person, hayfever will last for as long as you are exposed to the particular pollen to which you are allergic.

Food allergies: These have a wide variety of symptoms. The most obvious symptoms of an acute food allergy are a stomach upset followed quickly by nausea, vomiting or diarrhoea. People who are acutely sensitive to a food may also get a swollen tongue and lips. Sometimes the sufferer gets two kinds of symptoms; for instance, a child who is allergic to cow's milk may get diarrhoea and a skin rash. Apart from skin rashes, which may appear hours or even a few days after eating the food, these symptoms become apparent almost immediately after eating, usually within an hour. This makes it quite easy for the sufferer to identify the allergen.

Asthma attacks can also be brought on through an allergic reaction to foods and pollen, and this is characterized by wheezing, and difficulty in breathing.

Doctors now believe, however, that a variety of other physical and mental symptoms can be caused by food allergies though the cause can be difficult to identify. Depression, anxiety, headaches,

How allergy-producing histamine is released

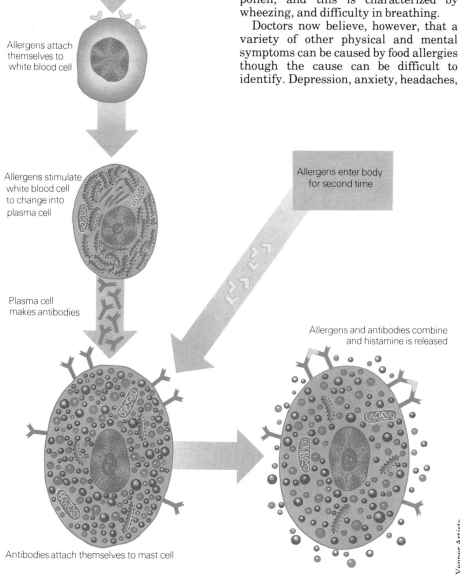

Allergen enters body

Allergens attach themselves to white blood cell

Allergens stimulate white blood cell to change into plasma cell

Plasma cell makes antibodies

Allergens enter body for second time

Allergens and antibodies combine and histamine is released

Antibodies attach themselves to mast cell

Venner Artists

Common allergies

Allergy	Allergen	Symptoms	Treatment	Prevention
Asthma	Dust mites Animal hair Pollen Some foods and food additives	Difficulty in breathing; wheezing	Prick test for diagnosis. Bronchodilator if breathing problem severe. Course of injections	Keep house dust-free. Avoid pollen; keep clear of allergic foods
Contact dermatitis	Contact with allergen, e.g. jewellery, chemicals in washing powder	Itchy, blistery inflammation	Steroid creams given on doctor's prescription	Avoid contact with allergen
Eczema	Some foods, especially cow's milk, flour, eggs; possibly some seafoods	Rash on hands face, neck, arms and legs; looks like scaly skin	Antihistamine tablets and creams given for skin condition	Take diet precautions to avoid allergen
Food allergy	Could be caused by almost any food—more commonly milk, flour, eggs; also strawberries, shellfish, nuts; some food additives	Upset stomach and general nausea; acute reaction produces swollen tongue and lips, as well as diarrhoea. If food is absorbed into bloodstream, it can produce skin rashes like eczema	Prick test. Elimination test. Provocation test for diagnosis of the allergen	Keep to diet; avoid allergenic foods
Hay fever	Pollen; may react to just one pollen or to several different types	Sore, itchy eyes, runny or stuffy nose, prolonged sneezing	Prick test to confirm allergy. Course of injections and antihistamine tablets to relieve symptoms	Course of injections before season begins. Listen to pollen count on weather report. Avoid open air. Wear dark glasses
Migraine	Usually caused by cheese, red wine, yeast extract, but not only caused by an allergy	Blinding headache	Elimination diet test if complaint due to food allergy	Avoid allergen foods
Nettlerash	Foods Handling certain plants Hot and cold water	Red, irritating swelling with with small white point in centre	Skin condition treated with with antihistamine cream, if necessary	Avoid the allergens

schizophrenia, hyperactivity in children and even convulsions have been attributed to food allergies. There have also been cases of bedwetting and cystitis which have been blamed on food allergies.

Migraine can also be caused by certain foods. Like yoghurt, chocolate, cheese, meat extracts, yeast extracts and some kinds of red wine which contain a substance called tyramine. Most people's bodies can deal with tyramine, which is not an allergen or poison in itself, but some migraine sufferers appear to lack a vital enzyme which breaks tyramine down. So when they eat these foods, tyramine builds up in their blood and sets off a chain of chemical events in the body which eventually results in the migraine headache.

Another complaint which is not strictly speaking an allergy but which is caused by food intolerance is coeliac disease. This is a disorder of the digestive system and its symptoms are wind and pain in the stomach after eating. Soft, smelly faeces (which are full of undigested fat) and weight loss, results from the sufferer's inability to absorb food properly. Coeliac disease is basically an intolerance of gluten, one of the proteins found in wheat. Sufferers therefore have to avoid foods which contain this substance.

The most severe—'though fortunately, quite rare'—symptom caused by allergy is anaphylaxis. In this instance, the patient's air passages swell and close and the blood pressure falls abruptly. This is an acute and life-threatening condition. though it can be reversed very quickly by an injection of adrenalin.

Causes
The basic difference between people who suffer from allergies and those who do not is still not known. Allergies do tend to run in families, and this may be due to an inherited characteristic in the cells which make up the immune system, which is the body's defence system against disease. But this is theory rather than proven fact.

However, it is known that most allergies are the result of an error in the immune system. The body's defence forces react to the allergen as if it were a dangerous infectious organism.

White blood cells called lymphocytes are one of the most important elements of the immune system. These cells are constantly on the look-out for foreign substances such as bacteria, viruses and proteins which are different from the body's own proteins and which may present a threat. When these white blood cells come across a potentially dangerous foreign protein they form a substance called antibody, which combines with the foreign protein and neutralizes it.

A slightly different antibody is created to deal with each foreign protein, but once it has been formed the body is able to produce it again to deal with any future 'attack' by that protein. This explains

Q I am worried that I may become addicted to the drugs I am using to treat an allergy. Could this happen?

A No. Nor do these drugs lose their effect if you have to keep taking them. However, they may have side-effects (antihistamines, for instance, can make you drowsy) and, like all drugs, should be treated with respect and caution.

Q Whenever my father is near my mother her eyes run and she can't stop sneezing. Can you be allergic to people, places or animals?

A No, you can't be allergic to a person, but there have been cases of wives who were allergic to their husbands' sperm. Some people who are acutely allergic to fish can get swollen lips from kissing someone who has just been eating fish. Allergy to animals is common, though it is the fine pieces of hair or fluff from the animal or bird which are to blame. You can only be allergic to a place if your are allergic to something found in that place – e.g. pollen.

Q I sit next to a girl in the office who has eczema and sometimes the rash is really bad. I can't help wondering if it is infectious.

A The simple answer is that allergies are not infectious. You cannot catch an allergy from another person, nor can you pick up a symptom – in this case eczema – of that allergy.

Q My husband and I have both suffered badly over the years from food allergies. Our two children have shown no signs of developing allergies, but we wonder whether they can be prevented.

A Some specialists say there is little that can be done, while others believe that some allergies can be prevented. The risk of becoming allergic to milk, for instance, may be reduced by breast-feeding rather than weaning on to cow's milk at an early age. Some specialists believe that you can reduce the risk of other food allergies by eating a more varied diet.

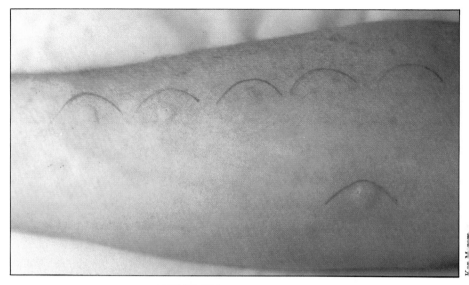

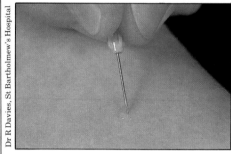

In the prick test, the skin of the arm is pricked several times and a drop of solution (see left) containing a possible allergen is dropped on to test for a reaction. This allergy sufferer (see above) has undergone the process and found that the cause of her allergy is the dust mite. The positive reaction to this allergen is shown in the large weal at the bottom. The marks above it show no reaction and represent negative results.

why we usually get infectious diseases like measles only once in our lives: after the first attack the body has supplies of antibody which can deal with the virus whenever it appears again.

By some highly complicated process, which is not yet understood by scientists, the immune system of a normal, healthy person knows how to tell the difference between a dangerous foreign protein (like a virus) and a harmless one, such as a food protein. But in an allergic person the immune system reacts to a harmless foreign protein as if it were a dangerous one, and starts forming an antibody. This antibody attaches itself to cells called mast cells. Mast cells contain a number of chemicals the most important of which is histamine.

When the body is exposed to the protein again, the antibody attached to the mast cells combines with the foreign proteins and tries to neutralize them. But in so doing it upsets the structure of the mast cell, which falls apart and releases its load of histamine. The surge of histamine produces an effect very much like the inflammation which follows a wound: it makes tiny blood vessels dilate, and as they dilate their walls become leaky, so that fluid from the blood escapes into the surrounding tissues. The dilation of the tiny blood vessels causes redness and itching, and the escaping fluid makes the

surrounding tissues swell. In hay fever the mucous glands in the nose and sinuses are also stimulated to produce fluid, which causes stuffiness and a runny nose.

Diagnosis

The diagnosis of pollen allergies (and sometimes of food allergies, too) is performed with the help of a technique called the prick test. The doctor or nurse gently pricks your arm with a needle, then drops a watery solution on the pricked spot. This solution contains a very small amount of one particular allergen.

Up to 40 of these little prick tests may be performed at one session without much discomfort for an adult. If you are allergic to one of the allergens, a round, red weal will show up on the spot within about fifteen minutes.

A special diet called the elimination diet is sometimes used to identify which food or foods are the cause of a food allergy. If you get better after being on this diet for several days, it is likely that one or more of the foods which have been eliminated will be the cause of your problems. You may then be asked to try these foods again to see if your symptoms return. This process of elimination is how the identity of the allergenic food is discovered.

As elimination diets can take a long time, some doctors now use provocation tests, in which a weak solution of various foods is either injected under your skin or dropped under your tongue to see if it will provoke symptoms. As well as testing for food allergies, the doctor may also test your reaction to chemicals which are commonly found in the home or used as flavouring, colouring or preservatives in food.

Treatment

If you have the acute kind of allergy which makes you sick whenever you eat say, strawberries or shellfish, you hardly need a doctor to diagnose your complaint. The cause and the effect are obvious, and the simplest way to deal with the allergy is to avoid the allergen.

Having discovered which pollen you are allergic to, the doctor may then prescribe a course of injections. These injections also contain small amounts of the allergen, and their aim is to desensitize you by encouraging your immune system to produce a harmless 'blocking antibody'. This kind of antibody intercepts the allergen before it sets off symptoms by alighting on the mast cell antibodies.

Courses of injections can be given during the pollen season, but this method is less reliable than giving the injections before the pollen season begins. These injections do not work for everybody, but they can give about 70 per cent of sufferers protection which lasts right through the summer.

Several kinds of drug are prescribed to deal with the symptoms of allergy. Antihistamines combat the inflammatory effects of histamine when it is released. They come as tablets, liquid medicine, nose drops or eye drops, and there are injectable antihistamines which can be used to deal with serious attacks. These drugs, however, do tend to make you feel drowsy.

Another drug, disodium cromoglycate (better known by its brand name Intal), works by preventing the mast cells from exploding. It therefore has to be taken before the symptoms occur; it can do nothing about histamine once it has been released. This drug can be given in the form of an inhalant (for asthma), eye drops (for allergic symptoms in the eye), tablets (for stomach allergies) or via another device called the insufflator, which lets you sniff it up your nose.

Corticosteroid drugs like cortisone, which are very powerful and anti-inflammatory, are sometimes prescribed for skin allergies or, via an inhaler, to combat asthma. Asthma can also be controlled by a group of drugs known as bronchodilators, so called because they dilate (open up) the bronchi (the air passages around the lungs).

It should be stressed that these drugs are not cures; they simply relieve the symptoms. Nor are they without problems. Corticosteroids have to be used sparingly and not for prolonged periods, and it is even possible to develop an allergy to antihistamines! It is important to let your doctor know if you are experiencing unpleasant side-effects from a medicine. There are many brands of anti-allergic drugs, and the doctor should be able to prescribe one which suits you better.

Food allergies can sometimes be relieved by drugs, but some doctors prefer to recommend diets which ensure that you eliminate all foods to which you have an allergic reaction.

Self-help

There is quite a lot that sufferers can do to help themselves. Obviously, if you suffer from a food or chemical allergy you should make every effort to avoid your allergens. This means that you should read the labels on food packets carefully to see whether the product contains even small amounts of the substance causing your particular allergy.

Hay fever sufferers should be careful about going out in the open air during the pollen season, especially in mid-afternoon when the pollen count is highest. Dark glasses can protect your eyes against pollen or spores, and it might be worth thinking about buying a small air conditioner for your home or car which can extract pollen from the air. Some cars now have filters in their ventilation systems which are designed to catch pollen before it enters the car.

If you are going on holiday in the late spring or early summer, bear in mind that there is usually much less pollen in the seaside air than in the middle of the countryside.

Dust mites are difficult to eliminate altogether from the home, but regular vacuum cleaning of carpets and curtains and washing of bedcovers will reduce their number. Artificial fibres in pillows and duvets are less likely to harbour dust mites than feathers.

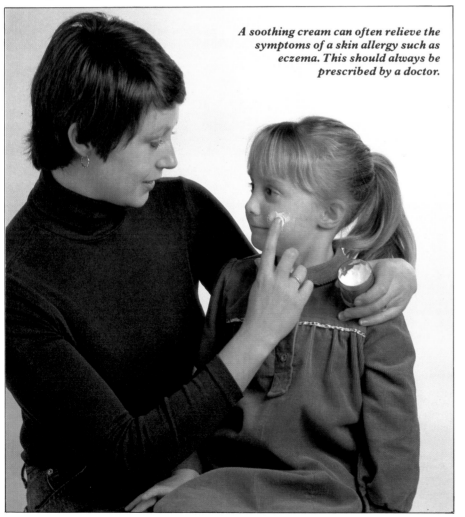

A soothing cream can often relieve the symptoms of a skin allergy such as eczema. This should always be prescribed by a doctor.

Amniocentesis

Is it too late for me to start a baby? I am 39 and this is my first marriage and we would so like a child.

A There is a good chance that you would have a healthy baby—and perhaps more than one—but don't fool yourself that there are no dangers. The risks of having a Down's syndrome child increases with the prospective mother's age, but luckily this condition can now be detected at an early stage of pregnancy. Do see your doctor and discuss the matter with him. He will refer you to a genetic counsellor if either of your medical histories show that this is a necessary precaution to ensure that you have all the information you need about any risks before becoming pregnant.

Q Do I have a choice about whether or not to have an abortion if amniocentesis shows that my baby is going to be abnormal?

A The decision is always left to the parents. You must imagine the life a handicapped child would have before deliberately bringing one into the world; and you should consider what would happen when you were no longer around to care for it. If you have strong objections to abortion on either moral or religious grounds, however, the final choice is obviously going to be even more difficult for you and you should discuss it with a professional counsellor or priest.

Q I'm so terrified that having a needle stuck into my tummy will hurt. But even more important, will it hurt my baby?

A You can be reassured on both counts. Before the needle is inserted into your abdomen, you will be given a local anaesthetic and will feel only a small pin-prick. Any discomfort is far more likely to arise from your reaction to this than from amniocentesis itself. As far as your baby is concerned, the whole purpose is to avoid injury. The needle is aimed carefully into the amniotic fluid and the ultrasound scanner will ensure that its insertion will be 100 per cent accurate

All mothers want their babies to be perfect, but until recently some mothers could not feel sure about this before the birth. Babies born to older women, or to those from families with inherited defects, were especially vulnerable. Now, with amniocentesis, medical science can help resolve these fears.

A diagnostic technique developed only in recent years, amniocentesis is used to check for abnormalities in unborn babies who may be at special risk. The test involves taking a sample of the amniotic fluid which surrounds the baby by inserting a hollow needle carefully through the expectant mother's abdomen. This may sound, and indeed look, unpleasant, but if skilfully done it does not even require an anaesthetic injection, though a local anaesthetic may be used.

The amount of fluid withdrawn is only about 20cc, the equivalent of two dessert spoonfuls, although this can vary according to the number of tests necessary. This fluid contains cells from the foetus (the developing baby). Chemical and microscopic examinations of these can provide invaluable information, revealing the presence or absence of genetic disorders, which at one time could only be guessed at, with often distressing results.

Defining a genetic disorder

The moment a human egg is fertilized, it has all the inherited information needed to create a new being. Both male and female cells contain chromosomes, which determine sex and carry the genes that transmit inherited characteristics, but occasionally these chromosomes are found to be faulty.

In the past, genetic counselling was very much a question of mathematics, of calculating the odds of a disease being passed on. Where both parents carried the same defective genes, for example, the risk of the disease was estimated at one in four; and if both parents actually suffered from the disease, instead of only carrying it, the odds were known to be even worse with the child almost sure of developing it.

When the test can be done

From about the 16th week, the doubts and fears which previously had to be endured throughout the pregnancy can be resolved. By this stage, there is enough amniotic fluid to allow the test to be carried out—and there is still time for the pregnancy to be terminated if this is thought to be necessary.

What it shows

The main disorders which amniocentesis can reveal are *spina bifida,* an abnormality of the nervous system where the baby either does not survive or is born with severe spinal defects, and Down's syndrome, which used to be known as mongolism. Examining the chromosomes can also reveal the sex of the baby, but the

Pregnant woman at 16 weeks

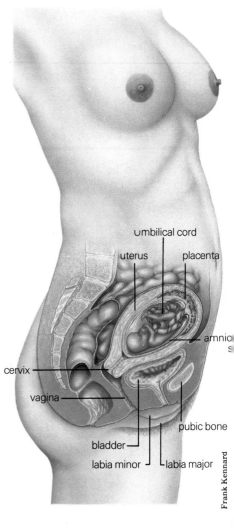

The sample of fluid from the amniotic sac is not taken until the pregnancy is advanced 16 weeks at the very earliest.

test is not done merely to satisfy curiosity without good medical reason. The sex of the baby only becomes medically important where there is known to be a history of a disorder such as *haemophilia* (excessive bleeding from the smallest wound) within a family. Although carried by females, the disease only affects males, and if the test reveals a male child a further test can confirm whether or not the baby is affected.

Ideally, amniocentesis should be offered to women over 35 because the risk of chromosome defects increases with age, although is is also recommended, regardless of age, to parents who have already had a baby with spina bifida, Down's syndrome or any rare defect which is detectable by this technique. As an example of how the prospective mother's age can affect the likelihood of having a defective child, the risk of Down's syndrome in babies born to women under the age of 25 is only one in 1,000 but rises to one in 40 for women over 40—and even more dramatically after that

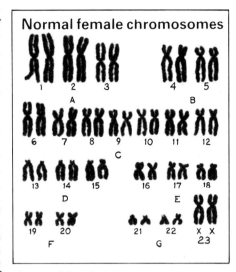

Normal female chromosomes

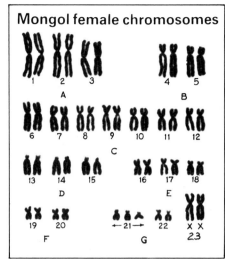

Mongol female chromosomes

A normal female child will have 23 pairs of chromosomes (above). Here (right), there is an extra number 21 chromosome. This is an abnormality and will result in a Down's syndrome child being born.

The risk to the baby

Amniocentesis is carried out quite simply in the outpatients' department of a hospital, with no risk to the mother-to-be but a slight possibility of risk to the baby. It is for this reason that the option to undergo testing is only offered; it is never imposed upon anyone.

About one in every 100 babies aborts after amniocentesis and, although many would have died or aborted anyway due to abnormalities, it still means that a few normal babies are lost. This is the risk that any pregnant woman who asks for, or agrees to, the test being performed must be prepared to face and accept from the beginning.

Fortunately, the technique of ultra-sound scanning is now used together with amniocentesis to give a picture of the position of the foetus in the uterus as the needle is inserted, so making the whole procedure very much safer for the unborn baby.

Making the decision

If a serious abnormality is found in the foetus, the parents are told and an abortion is offered to them. The final decision is always their own and some people may opt for termination rather than bring a seriously affected baby into the world.

While amniocentesis is vital in early pregnancy for detecting abnormalities, it also serves another very useful purpose late in pregnancy in that it can reveal valuable information about the develop-ment of the baby—aiding the doctors in their constant monitoring process.

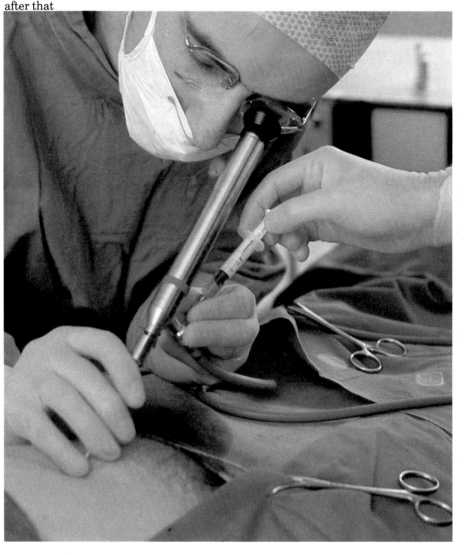

An even more advanced technique than amniocentesis is fetoscopy. A fetoscope (left) is inserted in the abdomen in a similar place as for amniocentesis and this allows direct viewing of the foetus to ensure normal development.

Amphetamines

Q Can you become addicted to slimming pills? My aunt tried some once—but they made her depressed and in the end she got fatter than ever.

A She may have taken an amphetamine-type drug to try to suppress her appetite. But these can only be given for short periods as they can have unpleasant after-effects. Nowadays, doctors agree that the best way to lose weight is to eat less. There are now safer substitutes that can be taken instead of amphetamines—if this is really necessary.

Q I'm keen on cycle racing. Can I take amphetamines before a race to improve my staying power?

A It is not safe to do so. In fact, it is on record that a professional cyclist taking part in the Tour de France race actually died from this. As a result, all national and international sports agencies ban the use of stimulants.

Q Our little boy seems to need less sleep than we do. He's still jumping around at two in the morning. Can we give him some pills to calm him down so that we can get some sleep?

A Absolutely not. Get some professional advice at once. Your doctor will advise you whether your child is really hyperactive or just needs very little sleep. You should never give a child pills without medical advice. Remember that a dose that has been prescribed for you will be much too strong for a child—it will do more harm than good.

Q I've missed money from my handbag and I suspect my 14-year-old daughter is taking it to buy drugs. Should I confront her about the matter?

A If you feel unable to speak to her about her problems, try and get her to talk to someone she trusts. Don't accuse her of stealing until you are quite sure of the facts. She may be suffering from adolescent depression and need all the help she can get.

Amphetamines are powerful, habit-forming stimulants which should not be taken unless medically prescribed. What, then, are the uses and abuses of these drugs?

When first discovered in the 1930s, amphetamine was hailed as a new 'wonder drug' because its stimulant effects bring such immediate and dramatic benefits: it increases mental alertness and physical stamina, relieves depression and acts as a slimming aid by suppressing appetite. But it was soon evident that its longer term effects were anything but beneficial, particularly because it was found to be habit-forming. Prolonged use requires larger doses and can result in serious psychological and physical conditions. Consequently, its medical uses are now strictly limited and it is now rarely given.

Pure amphetamine is a colourless liquid chemical from which several stimulant drugs are manufactured,

An over-active child is difficult for parents to cope with. It was found that medically supervised use of amphetamines was effective in such cases.

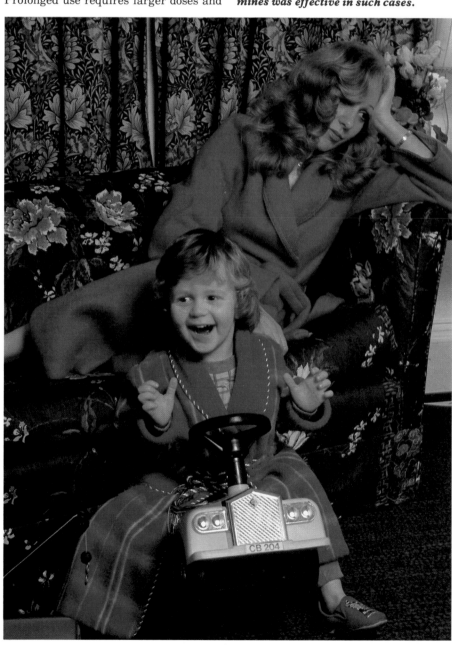

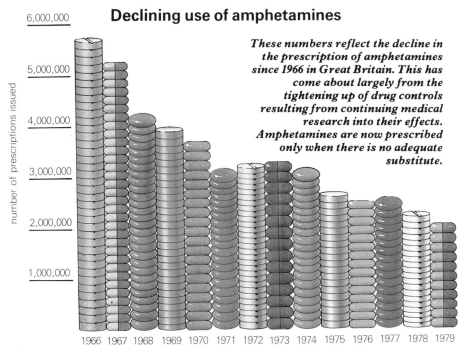

Declining use of amphetamines

These numbers reflect the decline in the prescription of amphetamines since 1966 in Great Britain. This has come about largely from the tightening up of drug controls resulting from continuing medical research into their effects. Amphetamines are now prescribed only when there is no adequate substitute.

usually in the form of tablets or capsules. Most commonly known are amphetamine sulphate (formerly sold as Benzedrine), the stronger dexamphetamine (Dexedrine) and methylamphetamine (previously marketed as Methedrine).

How it works

Amphetamine is chemically related to the body's own stimulant, adrenalin, and this enables it to mimic many of its effects. Adrenalin is released in the body in response to fear, excitement and physical activity. Both amphetamine and adrenalin prepare the body for what has been called 'fight or flight'.

The main action of amphetamine is to stimulate certain areas of the brain, so producing increased mental alertness, greater physical movement and more rapid breathing.

Even intelligence appears to improve — in fact, an average increase of eight points has been measured on the IQ scale. Through its influence on the nervous system, amphetamine produces other physical signs, like widening of the pupils of the eyes, and affects the normal movements of the intestine, stomach and bladder; the appetite also tends to be suppressed.

Medical uses

Amphetamine was first used in the treatment of an unusual condition known as narcolepsy, where the patient is constantly dropping off to sleep. This is still an accepted use today. In addition, it has been given for depression, Parkinsonism, epilepsy, and as a tonic and to counteract the depressant effects of barbiturate drugs and alcohol.

It has also been prescribed for bed-wetting and over-active children, because, paradoxically, it has been found to have a calming effect. However, it is important to remember that stimulants should never be given to children for this purpose unless prescribed by a doctor, and then only in the recommended dosage. This rule, of course, also applies to adult users who should know never to take drugs except on a doctor's order.

Slimming dangerously

In the 1950s, amphetamines were thought to cause little harm when taken as 'pep pills' and were also widely prescribed for women who had trouble in losing weight. Experience eventually proved that amphetamine-type drugs can only assist temporarily in the slimming process — none of the other effects are thought to be significant in helping weight-loss. Unfortunately, by the time the risks had been recognized, there were already thousands of patients dependent on them. It took some time for legal controls to be tightened.

The body does not become physically dependent on the drug, as it does with alcohol or barbiturates, but nevertheless, there can be serious psychological hazards if it is withdrawn suddenly. This 'let-down' effect shows itself in extreme fatigue, lengthy sleep and increased appetite. Another consequence of prolonged use which can be serious is listlessness and depression.

It has therefore become accepted that amphetamines should be used only for short periods in the treatment of obesity, taken in moderate doses and always combined with other measures, such as a low calorie diet. Some doctors take a stronger line and prefer not to use them at all for this purpose. There are now a great number of effective alternative appetite-suppressants in use which you can obtain on your doctor's prescription.

Drug abuse

In the 1960s, a new jargon and culture developed around the illegal use of amphetamines by youngsters who were often inadequate and insecure in other ways. 'Purple hearts' (which were, indeed, heart-shaped until the manufacturers changed their shape), 'bennies' and 'black bombers' were among the names given to those taken by mouth. 'Speed' was the name given to injected amphetamines and the user was known as a 'speed freak'. Obtaining them often involved theft or illegal manufacture and sale. This uncontrolled use had serious consequences for many young people whose health and lives suffered greatly as a result. This affected not only them, but their families and friends as well. In some cases the harm was long-term because of the disruption it caused at an important time of intellectual and emotional growth in their lives.

The risks of dependency

Those who become dependent on amphetamines are prone to accidents, they become aggressive and violent. They may have mental breakdowns, which result in delusions and hallucinations. Chronic amphetamine dependency can cause symptoms very similar to schizophrenia — an acute personality disorder often requiring hospitalization.

If an overdose has been taken, the signs in the victim are talkativeness, restlessness and trembling. Other signs are headache, flushing, irregular heartbeat, excessive sweating and stomach disturbances. In extreme cases, convulsions, unconsciousness and bleeding in the brain may occur.

To treat an overdose, the patient is given a sedative and a substance such as ammonium chloride which hastens the excretion of the drug in the urine.

Unfortunately, withdrawal cannot take place all at once, but must be carried out in gradual steps under professional supervision.

Perhaps the message that the uncontrolled use of amphetamines can be very dangerous is finally getting through. Certainly, their illegal use is declining and, hopefully, this will continue.

Anaemia

Q I am pregnant and seem to be getting paler and paler. Could I be anaemic?

A During pregnancy the body's demands for various essential nutrients, such as iron and folic acid, are increased. The developing foetus depletes the mother's natural store by absorbing them via the placenta, and this means the mother may become deficient. This can result in anaemia, unless extra supplies of iron and folate are given. Check with your doctor and, if you do prove to be anaemic, he will give you a prescription for the tablets you need to help you.

Q Can stress and strain cause anaemia? I have a very demanding job and seem to be continually tired.

A Anaemia cannot be caused by emotional problems alone; there is always an 'organic' basis. However, chronic depression, for instance, may be accompanied by a poor diet and this may eventually lead to anaemia through vitamin and iron deficiency. Have a chat with your doctor. You may simply be in need of a break.

Q I have heard that it is possible to prevent anaemia by the use of various tonics. Is this true?

A No. A normal diet, including meat, milk, fresh fruit and vegetables, will provide all the chemicals required to make blood. There is no benefit to be gained from tonics or vitamins bought over the counter.

Q My mother suffers from anaemia. I am worried that I or my children might have inherited it. Is this possible?

A Well, it depends on the type of anaemia in question. Some rare anemias such as Thalassaemia are passed on from generation to generation. In cases like pernicious anaemia the disease is not transmitted, but other family members are more likely to be affected. Common anaemias, like iron deficiency do not have a heritable basis.

People who look pale and feel run down often assume they are anaemic, but this is not necessarily so. And even if the condition is diagnosed, treatment is usually simple, quick and effective, giving a rapid return of health and energy.

Anaemia is the name given to a disorder of the blood, the composition of which is defective in some way. Usually it is the red blood cells that are affected. These are produced in the bone marrow, and contain an essential ingredient, haemoglobin. This substance has the remarkable ability to carry oxygen, which it picks up in the lungs and then distributes to the tissues of the body where it is needed to provide energy.

The marrow produces two million red cells a second and these survive in the bloodstream for about 120 days. If the level of blood cells in circulation is reduced from normal levels for any reason, this results in a lack of oxygen reaching the tissues and produces the classic symptoms of anaemia: a lack of energy, fainting fits, and skin pallor.

Causes

In general, anaemia is a superficial symptom of something else that is wrong in the body, and because of this there are a number of causes, the most common of which is a lack of iron. Iron is a mineral which is an essential ingredient of haemoglobin, as it is this that attracts the oxygen to the blood. When the supply of iron is reduced, the number of red blood cells in the body is also reduced and this leads to a shortage of oxygen.

This deficiency is often the result of eating the wrong foods, where the body is simply not being fed sufficient quantities of iron as part of the diet. It can also be caused by a severe blood loss. Women are particularly prone to this problem because of the amount of blood they lose each month during menstruation, a loss

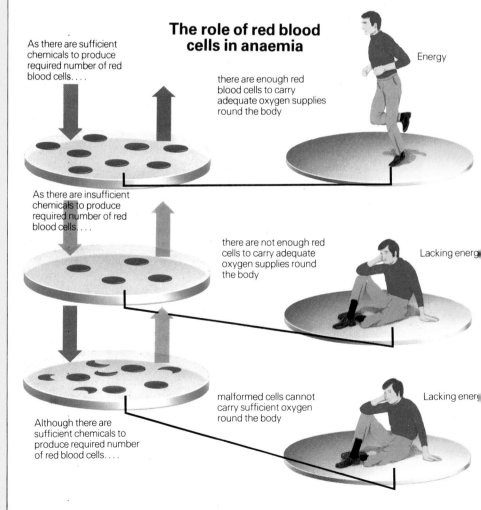

The role of red blood cells in anaemia

As there are sufficient chemicals to produce required number of red blood cells. . . .

there are enough red blood cells to carry adequate oxygen supplies round the body

Energy

As there are insufficient chemicals to produce required number of red blood cells. . . .

there are not enough red cells to carry adequate oxygen supplies round the body

Lacking energy

Although there are sufficient chemicals to produce required number of red blood cells. . . .

malformed cells cannot carry sufficient oxygen round the body

Lacking energy

Types of anaemia

Type	Causes	Treatment
Iron deficiency	Heavy menstrual loss; acute blood loss, bleeding duodenal ulcer; poor diet	Iron tablets or injections over several months
Pernicious anaemia	Failure of stomach lining to secrete substance called intrinsic factor	Vitamin B12 injections once a month for life
Anaemia of chronic diseases	Certain kidney diseases and some other chronic complaints	Anaemia usually disappears upon treatment of underlying disease
Aplastic anaemia	Bone marrow fails to make required number of red blood cells; can be brought about by cancer	Long-term; isolation; antibiotics and transfusions; drug treatment of bone marrow; bone marrow transplant
Sickle-cell anaemia	Defective red blood cells; genetic	If severe, transfusion; occasionally drugs
Thalassaemia	Defective haemoglobin; genetic	If severe, regular transfusions; occasionally removal of spleen (has no harmful effects)
Haemolytic (many types)	Red cells are killed off too early or in too great numbers in spleen	Drugs or removal of spleen, depending on type of anaemia.

that, if heavy, depletes the body of its store of iron. The problem also occurs during pregnancy when the mother loses iron during the development of the baby.

Further iron deficiencies are caused by peptic ulcers, where there is a slow but steady bleeding, and by parasites such as hookworms and tapeworms which feed off the blood.

Another condition known as pernicious anaemia occurs when the stomach lining fails to make and create a substance, imaginatively (if somewhat, confusingly) called intrinsic factor. This results in a deficiency of vitamin B12, a vitamin that is essential for the production of red blood cells. Since vitamin B12 can only be absorbed into the body with the help of intrinsic factor, if its secretion comes to a halt, the number of red cells is reduced resulting in an anaemic condition.

Chronic diseases, such as rheumatoid arthritis and certain kidney diseases, may also cause anaemia. The reason is not yet completely clear, but it appears that the body's ability to utilize iron breaks down.

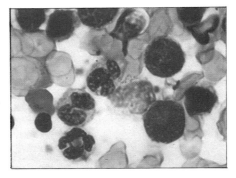

The larger, solid looking red blood cells in this bone marrow are typical of pernicious anaemia.

Instead of iron passing to the bone marrow, it is actually retained in the tissues. The resulting lack of iron in the marrow reduces the output of red blood cells.

A blood test used to diagnose the exact cause of the anaemia. A sample of blood is first collected from the patient (left) and then analyzed (right).

Perhaps the most serious form of anaemia is aplastic anaemia. This occurs when the bone marrow's ability to make red blood cells (as well as white cells and platelets—two further constituents of blood, both of which are made in the bone marrow) is arrested. Again, the cause is not fully known, but it does appear to be brought about by chemicals contained in some medicines or by cancer. This is a particularly unpleasant form of anaemia as not only do the body tissues lose their vital source of oxygen, but the body also loses the ability to ward off infection due to the lack of white cells.

There are many types of haemolytic anaemia, which occurs when the red cells are destroyed too quickly. It may occur either as a result of a blood transfusion mismatch or a complication with an Rh-negative mother. With some types of haemolytic anaemia there is a tendency to run in families.

There are further types of anaemia including those of a genetic and hereditary nature. Sickle-cell anaemia, common among black communities,

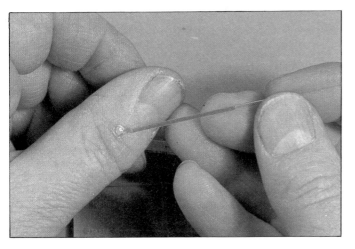

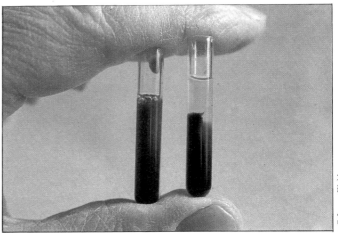

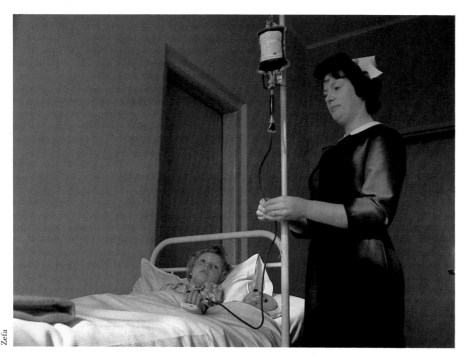

Zefa

arises through a malformation of the red blood cells, which fail to retain the necessary amount of oxygen. If severe, a blood transfusion may be necessary. Thalassaemia, common in Greek and other Mediterranean communities, is similar to sickle-cell anaemia but the haemoglobin is produced in an abnormal form.

Symptoms

To a great extent, the symptoms depend on the speed with which the anaemia develops, and this is influenced by the initial causes.

The most common symptoms are lethargy, pallor and breathlessness, sometimes accompanied by palpitations depending on the severity and type of anaemia. Severe cases of anaemia – such as those resulting from rapid loss of blood will cause fainting, dizziness and sweating. Symptoms of pernicious anaemia may also include 'pins and needles' in the hands and feet, nosebleeds, and, in extremely severe cases, heart failure.

When children suffer from iron deficiency they may also show signs of irritability and hold their breath. In severe cases of iron deficiency, the usual symptoms may be accompanied by jaundice, thirst, and some loss of control as the oxygen supply to the brain is reduced.

Aplastic anaemia can develop slowly, becoming obvious only weeks or months after exposure to a poison. It has all the normal symptoms of anaemia but is also accompanied by infections due to the deficiency of white blood cells.

If the anaemia becomes severe, a blood transfusion may be needed to ensure the necessary supply of oxygen to all parts of the body via the new blood.

Prevention

Most types of anaemia are impossible to guard against as they result from a malfunction of the blood-making system. But steps can be taken to prevent the onset of iron deficiency anaemia. Eating a good balanced diet of milk, meat (especially liver), fresh fruit and vegetables, all of which contain an abundant supply of all those vitamins needed to make blood and which are also rich in iron, will contribute to good health and keep anaemia at bay.

The modern fad of taking tonics and vitamin pills is of little or no value unless recommended by your doctor, or you have difficulty following a balanced diet. However, because of the demands made on their systems, pregnant mothers may be advised by their doctors to boost their iron intake with iron tablets.

Dangers

It is most important that the origin of the anaemia is diagnosed as soon as possible for a quick return to full health. With most forms of anaemia the dangers are not immediate, but the condition can deteriorate progressively if left untreated.

However, in the case of acute blood loss, if the condition is not promptly controlled it may lead to a fall in blood pressure and, in extreme cases, the resultant reduction in oxygen supply may be a threat to the person's life.

Chronic anaemia may often worsen an already existing disease, and this is particularly true of elderly patients.

Anaemia can be particularly dangerous during pregnancy, as it will be passed on to the child. This will deprive the child of the oxygen so necessary for growth and development.

Treatment

Treatments vary according to the anaemia, but invariably the patient will be treated to counteract the initial symptoms while undergoing tests to discover the underlying cause.

Simple iron deficiency anaemia is normally treated with a course of iron tablets or injections, often lasting several months.

With pernicious anaemia, the missing B_{12} vitamin has to be given on a regular basis – usually once a month. And since the cause of the missing vitamin is the stomach's failure to secrete the intrinsic factor – a disorder that will never improve – the treatment lasts for life.

Anaemia of chronic disease can only be treated by resolving the underlying disease. Once this is done the anaemia will disappear.

The treatment for aplastic anaemia is usually long-term, the patient being treated in a special isolation unit designed to prevent infection. The treatment consists of giving antibiotics by drip to fight infection, and regular blood transfusions to keep fresh blood in circulation. The patient's bone marrow may be encouraged to recover with the use of certain drugs. In some cases, bone marrow transplants have been very successful as a treatment for this type of complaint.

Outlook

This depends very much on the type of anaemia and on the presence of any underlying disorder. In some cases, such as pernicious anaemia, improvement can sometimes be dramatic.

Iron deficiency anaemia is usually cured fairly promptly with the patient gradually gaining in strength and energy. But the underlying cause will still have to be treated by drugs, diet or surgery.

The outlook for the sufferers of aplastic anaemia is not so good and bone marrow transplants are not an automatic cure in every case.

Nor are drugs always successful. However, doctors are hopeful of an improvement in the next few years.

In some cases of haemolytic forms of anaemia hospitalization may be necessary, but most types respond well to medical treatment.

Anaesthetics

Q I have heard that people can suddenly 'come round' on the operating table and know what is happening. Is this true?

A Provided the patient remains in the deeper stages of general anaesthesia, there is no 'coming round', although it is possible that the patient may dream that this is happening. Where an intravenous injection is used as the method of administering anaesthesia, it is possible for an unexpected 'coming round' to occur, but a skilled anaesthetist is always on guard against this.

Q My aunt told me that she was so nervous about a recent operation that she had to be given an injection before leaving the ward for the operating theatre. Why was this?

A This is quite usual and in no way out of the ordinary. All patients are usually treated to an appropriate 'cocktail' of drugs—called premedication—immediately before their operation. This makes the patients very drowsy and relaxed and also makes it much easier for the anaesthetist to do his job in the operating theatre.

Q Like most people, I have secrets that I do not want made public. I am very worried that I may talk when under a general anaesthetic. Is it likely that I may give away something that I may later regret?

A This is a common anxiety. When patients do mumble under anaesthesia, it is usually just dream-like nonsense. But in any case, the anaesthetist is a doctor and therefore bound by an oath of confidentiality with regard to what-ever patients may say. So you have nothing to fear.

Q Why do spinal anaesthetics work downwards and not upwards?

A Quite simply, the answer is gravity. If, for some reason, it is found to be necessary to affect the spinal cord above the site of the injection, the patient can be tilted to make it effective.

Anaesthetics are among the miracles of modern medicine. They ensure that otherwise painful treatments and operations are virtually pain-free. But how exactly does anaesthesia work?

In the days before anaesthetics even the most minor operation could be agonizing —early cartoons of people having teeth drawn without anaesthetic are enough to convince anyone of how fortunate we are today.

Modern anaesthetics can be divided into several different groups according to how and where they act to reduce pain. They can be given to patients in a number of different ways.

General anaesthetics

These are used in treatments and surgery where the patient needs to be completely unconscious. They are always given by a qualified anaesthetist, a medical doctor

The patient, having been taken from the ward, is being given oxygen prior to the injection of a general anaesthetic into his hand, immediately before being taken into the operating theatre.

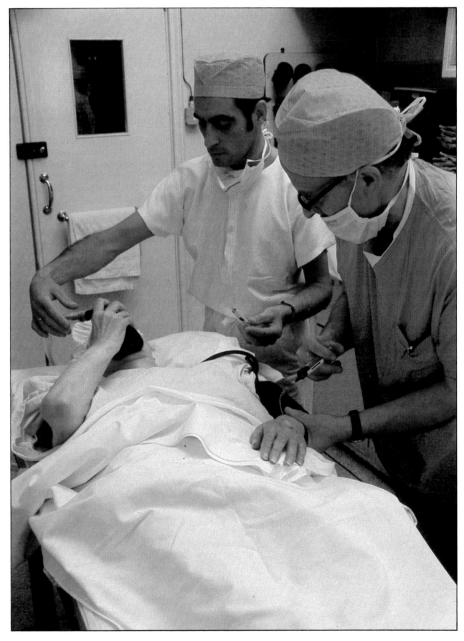

John Watney

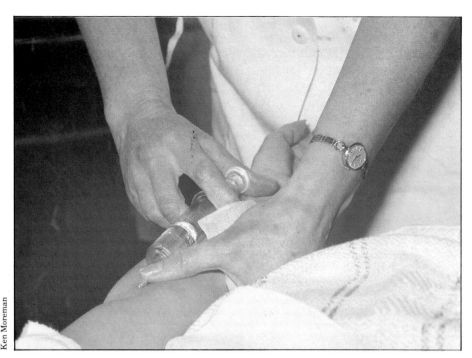

Ken Moreman

who has taken special training in the types and administration of anaesthesia. It is the anaesthetist's job to control the exact length of time during which the patient is to remain unconscious and to keep a careful watch on his or her physical condition.

They are given in one of two ways—either intravenously (injection into a vein) or by the patient's inhalation of a gas. Whether the injection is used on its own or combined with a gas at a later stage depends on the type and length of the operation.

Loss of consciousness may seem to occur quickly, but it is in fact a gradual process which happens in three different stages. In the first of these, the patient feels the pleasant sleep-like effects of the anaesthetic and starts to lose consciousness. This is the induction stage. The patient may feel extremely restless and talk aloud. During the second stage the patient is unconscious but still has some reflexes present and breathing is not quite regular. In the third and full stage of anaesthesia, the patient is fully unconscious with quiet regular breathing and relaxed muscles. The anaesthetist is trained to recognize the physical signs shown by the patient at each stage and ensure that any necessary action is taken. This continual monitoring is helped by the use of extremely sophisticated equipment in the operating theatre.

Many anaesthetic gases have been developed over the past 15 years, all of which are pleasant-smelling and ensure a quick return to consciousness.

When a general anaesthetic is given, muscle relaxants are also injected at the

A general anaesthetic may be injected into a vein in the arm, as shown here, or into the back of the hand as shown on the previous page.

same time. Their purpose is to ease the way into the anaesthetized state—and when muscles are relaxed medical investigations or surgery are much easier to carry out.

Local anaesthetics

These can be rubbed on the area in the form of ointment or swallowed—if an internal anaesthetic is needed—in the form of a gel. They can also be sprayed on, but perhaps the most usual way in which they are given is by injection, and many people are familiar with this use in dental treatment. They act by deadening the nerves in the area so that pain messages do not reach the brain.

They produce a numbing, freezing effect so that a surgeon can operate while the patient is fully conscious. The most widely used of the modern local anaesthetics is called lignocaine; it can be used in a variety of ways, but bupivacaine is a newer preparation with a longer-lasting action; this can be injected and is used as a spinal anaesthetic (an epidural) in childbirth.

Pain relief in childbirth

An epidural anaesthetic is injected into the epidural layer of the spine in the lower part of the back to numb a large area below the level of the injection. It affects the nerves which link the spinal cord and the womb, preventing pain messages from being transferred along the spinal cord to the brain. The needle is left in place, strapped to the woman's back, until the baby is born so that repeated doses can easily be given when necessary. This enables a woman to give birth painlessly while still conscious and able to co-operate where necessary, which is essential in childbirth. Epidurals are also used in gynaecological operations and, in

This inhaler allows the mother to breathe gas at her own rhythm to lessen the pain of contractions during labour. The gas is a mixture of one-half nitrous oxide and one-half oxygen.

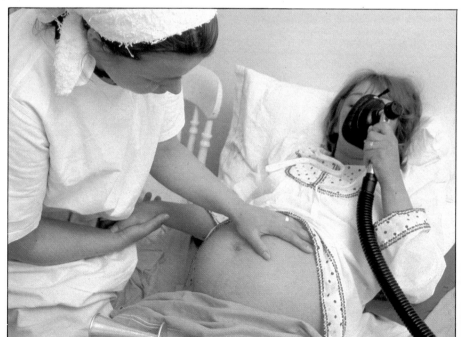

Types of anaesthetic

Anaesthetic	Effect	How given	Time needed to act
General	Complete loss of consciousness	Two methods: *Intravenous*—injection through a vein, usually at elbow or in hand (for shorter surgical or dental operations) *Inhalation*—given as gas through a mask (for longer operations or to maintain intravenous anaesthesia)	Rapid loss of consciousness. If patient told to count to 10—usually 'out' by number 7
Local	'Freezing' or numbing of particular area, e.g. gum and teeth in dentistry	Applied by spray or swab Made up in solution for injection or as drops As a gel or ointment	On surface—almost immediately Under skin—within minutes
Spinal (An epidural)	Gives pain relief without loss of consciousness — for childbirth, gynaecological or spinal operations	Injected into epidural layer of spinal canal	In minutes
Obstetric	Pain relief in childbirth without loss of consciousness. Slight drowsiness	Inhaled through mask held in hand. Automatically dropped when too drowsy	Only momentary loss of consciousness

Stages of general anaesthesia

Pre-medication	Stage One	Stage Two	Stage Three
A sedative injection is given to calm and relax patient while still in hospital ward. Can be combined with muscle relaxant injection	Pleasant sleep-like effect Loss of consciousness begins Some restlessness and talking aloud (Stage One is reached with gas and air pain relief in childbirth)	Patient is unconscious but reflexes still present Breathing not quite regular	Patient is fully unconscious Breathing is quiet and regular Muscles relaxed

some cases, it is used in the treatment of severe back problems.

There are other forms of pain relief available to women who decide not to have an epidural. To ease a painful contraction during labour, a woman can inhale gas and air (nitrous oxide with oxygen gas) using a vaporizer (a mask) which she holds in her hand. If she becomes too drowsy, she will automatically release the vaporizer; in this way she can have pain relief without completely losing consciousness.

For more difficult problems in childbirth, or for Caesarean birth, there are many modern general anaesthetics which can be used freely without risk either to mother or child.

Dental uses

Today, giving general anaesthetics during dentistry is losing popularity because of a number of fatal accidents which may have resulted because the dentist did not have the essential help of an anaesthetist. Any treatment requiring a general anaesthetic should be carried out in hospital—and many people now have their wisdom teeth removed under a general anaesthetic in hospital rather than in a dental surgery.

Local anaesthetics given by injection are still the most usual form of painkiller given, but many dentists are turning increasingly to the use of tranquillizers, such as Valium, especially in the case of more nervous patients.

After-effects

There are relatively few after-effects nowadays. With local and spinal anaesthetics, a little aching at the site of the injection may be felt for a few hours. In the case of general anaesthetics, the nausea and sickness that once occurred so frequently is now unusual. There may be some feeling of drowsiness, however, so that people who have had out-patient treatment or dental extraction should not drive a car immediately afterwards, and it is a wise precaution to see that there is someone to see them home.

Mild jaundice can occur, but this is a rare reaction to a general anaesthetic which should always be reported to the doctor immediately.

Anorexia nervosa

Q Sometimes I feel like going out and splurging on a bag of cream buns. Then I'm sorry, so I make myself sick afterwards. Am I anorexic?

A Not according to the actual definition of this illness. But watch out. You obviously feel guilty about overeating. Try to be less emotional about it and attempt to lose weight in a more sensible way.

Q Can anorexia occur in an older woman?

A Very occasionally. It is usually associated with immaturity, a fear of growing up, or the desire to revert to a child-like state, physically and mentally.

Q Are parents to blame for anorexia in a girl?

A Not in the deliberate sense. Girls with this problem often have very loving and protective parents. But sometimes this can be so repressive it stunts the normal process of growing up.

Q Can a person really die from slimming?

A Yes, if this turns into anorexia nervosa—from which about a quarter of the victims die. Fortunately, increased understanding and earlier treatment of this condition can give a better chance of a cure.

Q My friend has been told that she is anorexic, but she doesn't believe it. Why can't she realize how emaciated she looks?

A Because part of the disease itself is an abnormal mental state. A sufferer will look in a mirror but not see herself as she really is.

Q How is it that my daughter seems to eat normally but still loses weight?

A She may be pretending to eat but actually smuggling food out in her pocket or handbag. Suggest she sees the doctor to rule out any other cause of losing weight. He will understand the potential danger and take the necessary steps.

When a girl starts dieting, there may be more to it than a desire to be slim. Allowed to go too far, it can develop into anorexia nervosa—a potentially fatal disease. So it is vital for parents to know how they can help.

Anorexia nervosa is commonly known as the 'slimmer's disease', but despite this description its cause is far more complex than any simple desire to lose weight. It is also far more compulsive in its effects than ordinary slimming or dieting.

It almost always strikes young people between the ages of 11 and 30, and it affects more girls than boys. Apparently those from better-off homes are more prone to it than those from less affluent ones. This tends to suggest that anorexia nervosa is very much more a problem of the developed world.

Dramatic loss of weight is the obvious sign that something is wrong, and the person may need hospital treatment if it has reached a really serious stage. But, in the long run, the underlying causes must be diagnosed and remedied if treatment is to work and any improvement in weight and health maintained.

Causes

Once rare, anorexia nervosa is now tragically on the increase. The parents of victims may find it difficult to understand its cause, but more often than not the problem lies within the family. A daughter who never rebels or gives trouble, who delights her parents in every way and seems part of a perfect family, may

Teenage anorexics are often devious enough to hide food—something parents must be on their guard against.

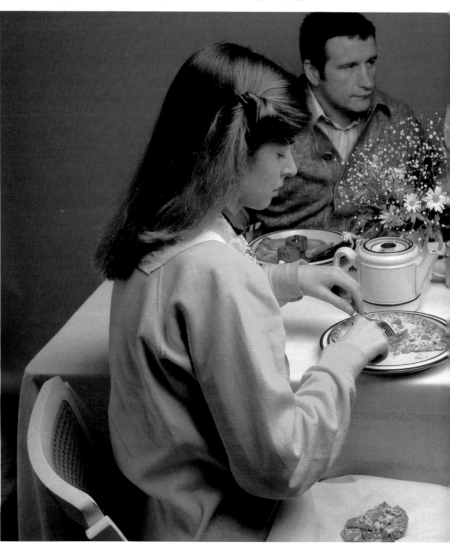

Di Lewis

secretly be tortured by a basic lack of confidence, self-esteem and a true idea of herself as a person. She may be too submissive and anxious to please for her own good. Her parents may have unwittingly been the cause of this situation by being over-protective, thus deterring her normal adolescent drive towards independence and a separate identity.

Behind such a girl's unexpressed feelings of inadequacy may lurk deeper and worse fears of the demands that maturity may bring. These can lead to thinness being seen as a desirable goal.

If body fat is made to disappear and a neutral childish figure retained, then the problems of adult life will not have to be faced. The popular image of slimness and superficial prettiness that is promoted by films, advertising and television may give a girl exactly the justification for which she is looking to account for her rejection of food. In fact, she may not be overweight at all.

Other girls diet drastically to increase their sexual confidence. These girls can

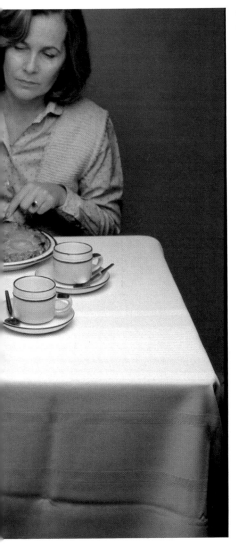

How to tell if your child is at risk		
Appearance	**Physical signs**	**Behaviour**
Haggard face	Periods cease	Hypersensitivity about appearance
Stick-like limbs	Diarrhoea, alternating with constipation	Food binges, followed by vomiting
Obvious loss of weight	Vomiting	Smuggling food away; pretending to eat
Clothes too big	Cold skin	Undue interest in and purchasing of laxatives, emetics, diuretics and enemas
	Poor circulation	Bad results from school
		Anti-social acts, e.g. stealing or deliberately breaking things
	Liability to infection	Withdrawal from friends

obstinately cling to the distorted idea that their extreme emaciation is beautiful, ignoring the harrowing evidence to the contrary which is only too obvious to everyone else.

Dangers

Experience has shown that the more distorted an idea the victim has of herself, the more difficult the cure, and the longer the condition goes untreated the more uncertain the outcome. In the past, death rates of between five and 25 per cent have been reported, but better understanding of the causes may improve the situation.

Anorexia nervosa must never be lightly dismissed as a passing fad or phase, which time and maturity will cure. The anorexic is *not* mature, nor is she suddenly likely to become so. Spontaneous cures rarely happen because the victim takes a positive pride in sustaining her hunger strike.

The longer the illness lasts and the more weight that is lost, the greater the sense of achievement. This deepens in the anorexic the illusion that being thin is making her significant and outstanding as an individual. In more real terms it is also succeeding in focusing attention and at last providing a form of personal rebellion against parental authority that should have been made much earlier—and in a less dangerous form—as part of growing up.

Compulsive dieting

When a normal person embarks on drastic dieting they can stop when they so choose. Most find it so unpleasant to be hungry or deprived of favourite foods in the midst of plenty, that the real problem is keeping to the diet. But the anorexic,

once set on a course of self-starvation, cannot go into reverse. It is as though they are the victims of a feeling not unlike that imposed by alcohol or drugs—and with something of the same lightheadedness.

It has been suggested that anorexics may even have a different body chemistry, but this has never been proved. It seems far more likely that they simply have a different mental outlook and confused motives that can involve not only self-punishment but also punishment of their parents.

Symptoms

It is vital that the illness is recognized and that treatment started as early as possible. This is not easy in the initial stages until the weight loss becomes so obvious that it is clear that something is severely wrong and a visit to the doctor really necessary. An unmistakable symptom in a girl, once weight has fallen below 46kg (103 lb) or thereabouts, is that her periods stop.

It may be discovered that she is making herself vomit, either to get rid of food she has been coaxed to eat or as part of a 'binge-and-vomit' pattern, enabling her to indulge in food without putting on the detested weight. In the end, the body becomes so accustomed to existing on a greatly reduced amount of food, that it has difficulty in coping with a large meal.

In a few cases, anorexics use emetics, laxatives, diuretics and even enemas, and over a period of time they can badly disturb body chemistry and greatly increase the risk of a fatal outcome. Obviously, prolonged starvation can mean a general weakening in victims and a greater susceptibility to infection.

Q My new boyfriend says that I'm too fat! In fact, I've always tended to be overweight and would like to do something about it—but I'm worried that I might overdo things and even develop anorexia nervosa and become really ill.

A Anorexia nervosa is not something that you catch, or that steals up on you in the night! Although it is the result of excessive or crazy dieting that pays no attention to the body's basic needs, it is fundamentally due to a disordered state of mind with regard to weight in particular and the rest of life in general. If you use a scientifically worked out diet—one that will enable you to lose weight but that still ensures that you get enough of all the food substances that your body cannot do without—you will never be in danger of getting anorexia nervosa. And you will be able to become as slim as you decide is best for you in perfect safety!

Q My grandmother, who is seventy-two, was in hospital recently for some tests and overheard the specialist say to his students that she had anorexia. I thought that this only happened to people of my age or am I completely wrong?

A There is a confusion of terms here. The anorexia you have in mind, which most commonly occurs in adolescent girls and which has been very much on the increase in recent years and consequently very much on people's minds and in the news is strictly speaking called anorexia nervosa, although it is often referred to as anorexia for short. But anorexia as a medical term has been around for centuries. It means loss of, or poor, appetite and is usually acccompanied by loss of weight—and it was most likely this that the specialist meant when he was discussing your grandmother's case with his students.

Anorexia is an important feature in many conditions such as alcoholism, anxiety states and cancer. These possibilities are all carefully considered by the doctor when a case of suspected anorexia nervosa is being investigated to determine the best treatment.

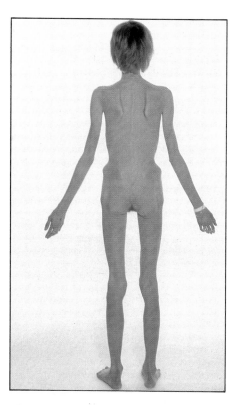

This anorexic girl, aged nineteen, was admitted to hospital and placed under treatment.

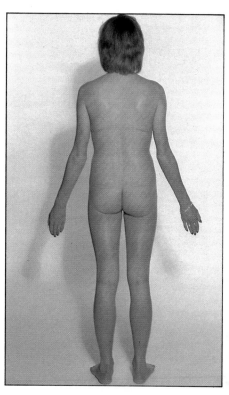

Two months later, she had returned to her normal body weight and had established good eating habits.

Treatment

Alert families should call for medical help long before symptoms are acute. The first job is often to restore weight to at least above danger level, before psychiatric treatment can commence. American research on this condition suggests that there is a critical weight which must be achieved, between 41 and 43 kg (90 and 95 lb) before psychotherapy can penetrate the strange mental isolation that starvation imposes and allow real communication to take place.

Weight gain for the anorexic often requires a prolonged stay in hospital, with intravenous feeding in the early stages. To coax the patient gradually to eat normal food and gain a set amount of weight, a system of rewards and withdrawal of privileges has been widely used. The basis for rewards is often a list drawn up by the patient and includes such things as being allowed to get up to go to the toilet, having extra visitors, wearing day clothes, going home on leave or, finally, going home altogether.

Maintaining a successful weight increase at home is made difficult by the extreme cunning of anorexics, who will use fair means or foul to avoid eating. They will deceive parents into believing they are eating a main meal at school or at work, and at home will toy with food, pretending to eat while secretly smug-gling it from the table in pockets or handkerchiefs. They have even been known to fake a weight gain on the scales by putting weights in their pockets.

In a hospital ward, of course, this type of deception is less easy; weight is monitered and bed rest imposed. Also, in the early stages, a tranquillizer may be used. This will be given intravenously, if necessary, for those patients who know how to induce vomiting when given drugs or food by mouth.

Future action

Once enough weight has been gained for the patient to be out of immediate danger, the more difficult part of the treatment can begin. This will include some family counselling, so that parents can understand the nature of the illness and its causes and so learn to cope with it.

Initially, the victim has to be convinced that anorexia nervosa is not just a matter of weight loss. The girl, helped by the therapist, can then begin her own search and fight for identity, dealing with the inner doubts and fears that plagued her, accepting the challenges and appreciating the real promise of her own sexuality and maturity. She must be helped to realize that her old ideas about herself were distorted and to replace them gradually with a truer picture. With this will come the self-confidence to grow up.

Antenatal care

Q Years ago, I thought I had VD but never went for a check-up. Now I am pregnant and feel so worried that I may have passed it on to my baby.

A There is no need to feel anxious about this. If you had contracted VD at any stage, it would have shown up in the tests made during the routine of your antenatal care. You would have been told if you had anything to worry about.

Q I have been told that I should scrub my nipples with a nail brush to prepare them for breast feeding. I have tried to do this but it is very painful. Is it really necessary?

A No, certainly not. You need only moisturize your breasts in the same way as the rest of your body, and wear a good bra. If you have inverted nipples (i.e. they do not stick out enough), however, ask your doctor for advice, as there could be problems with breast feeding.

Q Is it possible to establish the sex of my baby before it is born. And if so, how?

A A test called amniocentesis can be carried out to show the sex of your baby. However, it is only run when there is a suspicion that the baby is abnormal—and it does carry a small risk. It is therefore unlikely that you will be able to take the test to identify sex only. And anyway, surely part of the fun of having a baby is *not* knowing the sex it is?

Q Is it dangerous for my husband and me to make love? I am in my eighth month of pregnancy.

A If you and the baby are in good health, there is no reason at all why you should not continue your lovemaking until the very end of your pregnancy. In fact, it is probably very good for your relationship at this important time. And if you have problems finding a comfortable position, try something new— preferably where penetration is not too deep. Of course, should there be any discomfort, pain or bleeding, you should see your doctor at once for a checkup.

If you are an expectant mother, it is of vital importance to stay fit and well throughout your pregnancy, and so help to ensure having an easy birth and a healthy baby.

Every year in Great Britain, 15 babies out of 1000 are either stillborn or die within one week of their birth. But many of these deaths could have been avoided if mothers had taken advantage of the antenatal care facilities available. This involves regular visits to the doctor, a balanced diet and controlled daily exercise and rest.

Diet and general health

A well balanced diet is essential during pregnancy. 'Eating for two' is unnecessary. In fact, gaining too much weight is bad for both mother and baby and makes it more difficult for you to regain your figure after the birth. The total weight gain during pregnancy should not be more than between 12-14 kg (25-28 lb). What is important is to ensure that you get the best nutritional value from your food and eat in sensible quantities.

Your daily diet should include protein—two or three helpings of meat, fish or cheese; milk—half a litre (one pint); vegetables and salad—two helpings; fresh fruit—two portions, to include one citrus fruit or its juice; butter or margarine in moderation; wholemeal bread—four to five slices (or substitute cereal or pasta for some of the slices).

Vitamins play an important part in our general health and are easily absorbed through sensible eating. Routine 'multi-vitamin' supplements during pregnancy are unnecessary, unless your doctor finds otherwise.

Minerals are as important as vitamins to the pregnant woman. They are also readily available in the foods we eat. Most hospitals distribute iron tablets as a routine measure during the last three months of pregnancy. Calcium is also often given as a supplement.

Helping yourself

Though pregnancy is certainly not an illness, many women do suffer from minor ailments which can make them miserable. Many of these can be avoided by knowing how to take care of yourself.

If you suffer from nausea and vomiting—eat a dry biscuit with tea before getting up in the morning. It helps to eat little and often.

To prevent indigestion and heartburn, avoid fried foods and try not to eat too late at night; allow plenty of time to digest food before going to bed.

Backache can be a problem, so pay special attention to posture; avoid picking up or carrying heavy items.

To avoid constipation and the possibility of piles, include roughage in your daily diet—vegetables, fruit, wholemeal bread, bran and cereal. Drink six to eight glasses of water a day and take gentle

A sensible, well balanced diet is essential to the health of both mother and baby. Two portions of fresh fruit daily, including citrus fruit, are recommended.

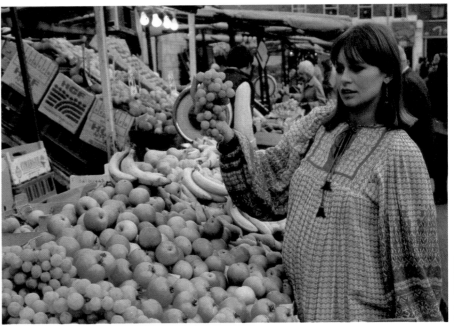

Anthea Sieveking

exercise, such as walking or yoga.

To prevent varicose veins getting worse, wear support tights and avoid standing for too long at a time. Prop up your feet whenever you can.

Avoid trouble with your teeth by spending more time on dental hygiene and massaging your gums. Do not eat decay-producing sweet foods.

Finally, guard against any risk to the developing foetus. Try to stop smoking and limit drinking alcohol—both are potentially harmful. And if you are taking medication of any kind, check that this is safe.

Medical care

As soon as your pregnancy has been confirmed, discuss with your doctor where you are going to have the baby—in hospital or at home.

Home deliveries are often difficult to arrange. They are only possible if your medical and obstetric history is favour-able and the facilities at home are satisfactory for the care of both mother and child.

If your baby is going to be born in hospital, there are several points that are worth checking. Ask whether your partner can be present at the birth, and if you will be allowed to do exercises, which may involve getting up and walking around during labour. You should find out what type of pain relief is used or if a choice is available. Most expectant mothers will also want to know if they can keep their babies with them after the birth and the hospital's attitude to breast feeding.

The waiting months

Antenatal clinics are usually attached to a hospital, or your own doctor may pro-vide antenatal care.

The first visit should be made between the first eight to 12 weeks of pregnancy. The doctor will check your medical history, including details of previous pregnancies, any hereditary illnesses and the general state of your health.

He or she will then give you a general examination and measure your weight, height and blood pressure. You may have an internal examination. Samples of urine and blood will be taken for tests, and a card detailing your medical history, the tests carried out and the progress of the pregnancy may be issued.

Your next visit will be four weeks later, and then at four-weekly intervals up to the 28th week of your pregnancy. After that, you will need a check-up every two

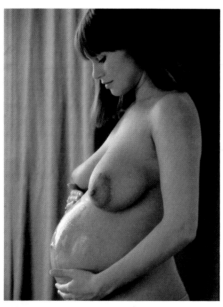

Skin care is important in pregnancy. To help prevent stretch marks massage oil into your breasts and abdomen.

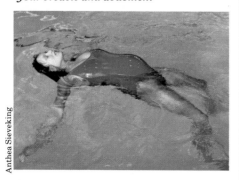

Anthea Sieveking

Deep relaxation can be practised while floating on your back. Or lie in bed and allow your body to 'let go' completely.

Exercise and posture during pregnan

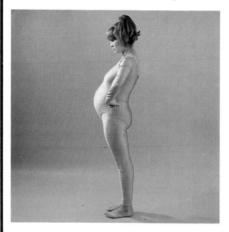

Incorrect standing posture: avoid the natural tendency to compensate for the extra weight by leaning backwards.

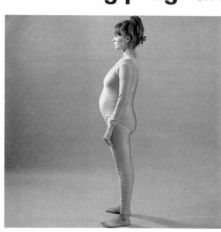

Correct standing posture: stand straight with shoulders relaxed and abdomen and bottom tucked in.

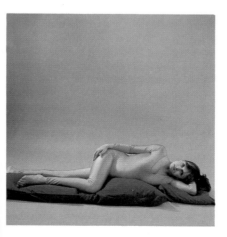

In late pregnancy many women prefer to sleep lying on their side. A cushion between the legs gives extra comfort.

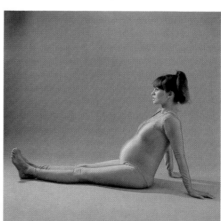

In this position practise tensing and relaxing the muscles around the anus and around the vagina and urethra.

weeks up to the 36th week, then every week until the baby is born. If there are any problems, more frequent visits may be necessary.

Each time, you will be asked how you feel, have a urine test, your blood pressure and weight will be checked and your abdomen examined. The doctor will listen to the foetal heartbeat and you may have an internal examination.

There will also be discussions on the emotional and physical problems that occur in pregnancy, and the emotional reactions which may be experienced after the birth. Advice on breast feeding or bottle feeding is given. You will also be shown exercises that will help you to regain your figure after your baby is born.

Expectant fathers are also taught about pregnancy and advised about helping at each stage.

Physical preparations
One of the commonest problems throughout pregnancy is bad posture. Try standing, walking and sitting properly; it will soon come naturally.

The three main exercises to practise are the pelvic floor and abdominal exercises and the birth position.

There are various relaxation techniques that you can perfect. Conscious relaxation can be practised at any time; check that your facial muscles, shoulders and hands are not tense. Relax by dropping your shoulders and unclenching your hands. Disassociation relaxation is a particularly good technique to learn for coping with labour. This involves tensing one set of muscles while keeping the remaining muscles in your body relaxed. Deep relaxation is best practised before going to sleep. Lie down comfortably and allow your body to 'let go'.

There are three basic breathing levels which can be used during labour. The principle to be followed each time is to avoid holding your breath and to 'go with' the contractions.

The first level can be used throughout labour, but it is especially good in the early stages. It involves deep abdominal breathing. Breathe in deeply, using your abdomen on the 'out' breath.

The second and third levels are generally used when the contractions are stronger. For second level breathing, take a shallower breath and place the emphasis on the 'out' breath. For the third level, breathe in and out very gently, again with the emphasis on the 'out' breath.

Huffing and puffing is useful in the stage of labour just before the cervix (neck of the womb) is fully dilated. It involves taking two shallow breaths while still emphasizing the 'out' breath each time, then blowing 'out' quickly twice. The breath should be allowed to flow back into the lungs each time.

Also practise gentle panting through the mouth; this is used to help stop pushing as the baby's head is 'crowning', i.e. the outer lips (vulva) are fully dilated round the head.

Massage can be of great help during labour. Back massage is good for backache and also gives considerable relief if contractions are felt in the back. Leg massage is helpful against cramp.

Yoga and stretching exercises can be of great benefit to us all, but especially if

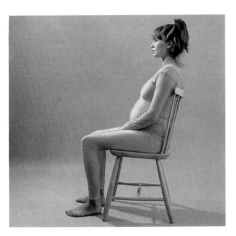

Sit comfortably, in a relaxed position, with your back straight and supported by the back of a hard chair.

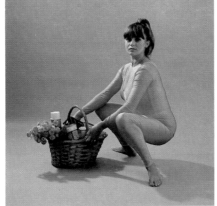

In lifting an object keep back straight and bend from the knees. Avoid bending over, which strains muscles.

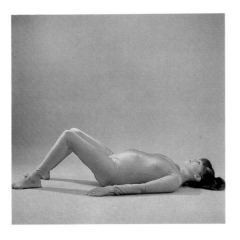

For abdominal muscle tone; lie on floor as shown, tighten abdomen, pulling baby towards the backbone.

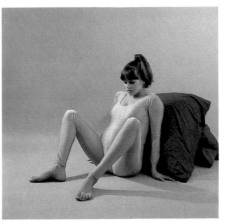

Assume delivery position, as shown, with back at 45° angle. Tense and relax pelvic floor and thigh muscles.

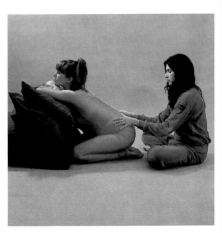

Back massage will help during labour, relieving backache and contractions if they are felt in the back.

Q I am a twin and my husband's family also has a history of twins. I am now 12 weeks pregnant and am wondering how soon I can find out whether I am going to have one child or more.

A Sixteen weeks is the earliest that you can be sure of clear results from an ultrasound scan, which many hospitals run as a matter of routine at this stage. If this is not the case with your hospital, tell them of your concern and they will arrange a test for you.

Q I have a very small frame and my baby is thought to be very large. My doctor wants me to have an X-ray to establish the size of my baby's head in relation to my pelvis. Won't this damage my unborn child?

A The doctor will not take the X-ray until the last four weeks of pregnancy. It is in the first three months that the foetus is most vulnerable and likely to be damaged by the rays. This applies to X-rays on any part of the body; so remember to tell your dentist that you are pregnant if he or she decided to X-ray your teeth. X-rays are hardly ever used on expectant mothers these days; the ultrasound scan is considered sufficient in most cases. However, there are exceptions, such as in your case, when there is doubt about the size of the pelvis, the baby is incorrectly positioned or if the baby is upside down and a breech birth is expected.

Q My husband and I both feel it is important that he should be present at our baby's birth. Is this possible?

A Most hospitals welcome the presence of the father at the birth, but check that this is so in your case. Many antenatal classes also involve the expectant father, preparing him to help during the labour rather than just watch. The midwife may allow your husband to help you give birth by holding up your legs and putting an arm round you to support your back. He can also guide you through your contractions if you are using relaxation techniques. And both of you can benefit from sharing the moments following birth.

Tests you may be given

Test	How often	Reason
Urine	Each antenatal visit; occasionally a 24-hour sample is collected	To check sugar and protein levels; to check hormone level to see if placenta, which links mother and baby, is functioning correctly
Cervical Smear	Once	Cells are analysed to see whether there are any infections, such as gonorrhoea or thrush, or early pre-cancerous changes
Blood tests	First antenatal visit	Blood group is established and checked for anti-bodies that could affect the baby; haemoglobin level for anaemia; venereal disease; susceptibility to German measles
	16-17 weeks	Defects in baby, such as anencephaly; other neural tube (the tube enclosing spinal fluid) defects
	Subsequent	Anaemia, if condition is suspected on first visit
Ultrasound Scan	At 16 weeks (routine at some hospitals)	Establishes size of baby; measures foetal heart beat. It has largely replaced X-rays as a way of monitoring a baby's development. Can confirm number of babies in uterus)
Amniocentesis	Rarely	The mother is over the age of 35 or there is a suspicion of an abnormality such as Down's syndrome, spina bifida or other neural tube defects

you are pregnant. Practise every day for at least four months before the birth. They will help relaxation and strengthen the muscles used for childbirth.

Taking care of your appearance
If you look good when you are pregnant, you will feel good. Always wear comfortable clothes, in flattering colours. Never wear clothes that are too tight and remember that properly fitting underwear is very important, especially a good maternity bra. Wear shoes that are comfortable, low heeled or flat, and if you have varicose veins, always wear support tights. Keep your hair in good condition.

Pay special attention to your skin as part of your daily routine. Use moisturiser on your hands, neck and face. Pour a little baby oil into your daily bath, and massage oil into your breasts and abdomen. This helps prevent stretch marks.

Finally, practise antenatal and breathing exercises for ten minutes each day and rest to build up reserves of energy.

Antenatal classes
By the 20th week of your pregnancy you should enrol in an antenatal class. These classes are run by hospitals, the social services and private and charitable organizations.

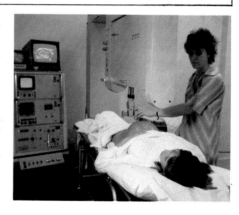

An ultrasound scan provides a picture of the foetus (on the screen), enabling the doctor to determine its exact age.

In these classes the growth of the foetus in its various stages will be explained. You will also be shown exercises that aid relaxation, help prevent physical problems and prepare the muscles that will be used in labour.

Next, you will be told about the whole process of birth and you may be shown a film of an actual delivery. You will also learn about labour and what to expect at each stage, various delivery positions, analgesics (painkillers), and how to breathe correctly.

Your nutritional needs during pregnancy

Nutrients	Sources	Effects
Proteins	Meat, fish, poultry, dairy products, dried beans, peas, pulses, nuts, grains and some vegetables	Build the tissues that form the baby, aid the growth of the placenta and help strengthen the uterus
Carbohydrates	Flour, cereals, fruit, starchy vegetables, honey and milk	Energy producing foods which, if taken in excess, cause obesity. Most women, however, need more calories than usual during pregnancy
Fats	Meat, poultry, oily fish, dairy products, eggs, oils and nuts	Fats are necessary to a balanced diet because they help the body absorb vitamins. But be careful, they can easily cause obesity
Vitamin A	Dairy products, fish liver oils, margarine, oily fish offal, carrots, apricots, tomatoes, green vegetables	Good for the skin, eyes, bones and many of the internal organs
Vitamin B Group	Green leafy vegetables, wholewheat products, liver, kidneys and brewer's yeast	Help prevent constipation, nervousness, skin problems, increase the energy level and help form red blood cells
Vitamin C	Citrus fruits, berry fruits, green vegetables, salad vegetables, peppers, parsley, tomatoes and potatoes (but remember that overcooking destroys the vitamins)	Strengthens the placenta, aids the absorption of iron and helps in the formation of the baby's skin, ligaments and bones
Vitamin D	Fish liver oils, oily fish, margarine, eggs, butter, cheese, liver	Helps the body absorb calcium which is essential to build and strengthen bones
Vitamin E	Apples, carrots, cabbage, celery, eggs, muesli, olive oil and sunflower seeds	Helps circulation
Vitamin K	Green leafy vegetables, eggs, cereals, potatoes, strawberries	Important in the development of the blood clotting process
Calcium	Dairy products, fish, nuts, oranges, raspberries, dried fruit, leafy green vegetables, swedes, turnips, cauliflower and sesame seeds	Builds the bones and teeth of the growing baby
Iron	Meat (especially offal), cereal products, eggs, pilchards, sardines, spinach, parsley, watercress, cocoa, chocolate, black treacle and nuts.	Prevents anaemia—the baby has to store a reserve of iron in its liver on which to draw while being on a milk diet after birth. It continually saps the mother's natural supply in the womb which makes supplements necessary

Yoga exercises

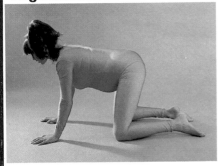

All fours position: start by sitting on your heels; bend forwards onto knees; keep back straight, as relaxed as possible.

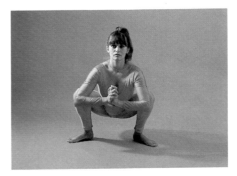

Squatting: start in a standing position, legs apart, then squat. This helps prevent backache and constipation.

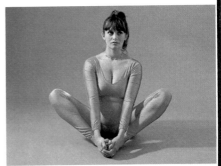

The tailor: sit upright, on front of buttocks. Gently push knees down with elbows; lift thighs and lower them.

Anthea Sieveking

Anthrax

Q My husband is a dock worker and I can't help worrying about him catching something horrible from the cargoes he handles. Could this happen?

A Don't worry. The likelihood is minimal. Port authorities everywhere are aware of the precautions which must be taken to prevent any risk of contact with infected animal products. In this case, masks and protective clothing must be worn and hygiene measures rigorously observed.

Q My hobby is collecting and spinning wool. Is it possible to contract anthrax from this?

A This is unlikely in a country where the disease does not occur on any scale. Home wool spinners have little to fear, provided they know the farms from which they collect their wool. But, should wool be collected from an infected animal, there is every risk that it may contain anthrax spores. Indeed, among people who handled wool in their jobs in the past, anthrax was known as 'woolworkers' disease'. So if a case of anthrax has occurred in your area, it is wiser to stop wool-gathering trips.

Q Could anthrax bacteria be used in germ warfare? And is there any protection against this?

A Regrettably, the bacteria could be used in germ warfare to cause anthrax of the lungs, and the chances of survival would be remote. Protective measures would be impracticable against such a fearful 'weapon'. Unfortunately, mankind now has almost unlimited means of self-destruction—either by mechanical or bacteriological means. The moral implications of this are a matter of international and humanitarian concern.

Q Can you tell me why the lung form of anthrax infection is usually fatal?

A Because infection of the lungs spreads directly into the bloodstream, unlike the skin variety of infection. This mean that a fatality is more likely unless treatment is immediate.

Anthrax is a virulent infection which medical researchers are working towards wiping out completely.

Anthrax is caught from diseased animals. It can affect goats, cattle, sheep and horses, causing sudden death. In humans, it produces a slowly progressive skin condition, or a rarer lung infection, which can be lethal in 90 per cent of the cases.

Anthrax is caused by the growth and spread of a bacterium—*bacillus anthracis*—capable of lying dormant as spores. It can survive heat, cold, drought and most disinfectants. The spores can be carried in animal products such as skins, hair, fleece and bonemeal, and this makes humans easily open to infection. If a spore penetrates the skin via a tiny wound or is inhaled the bacteria begin to breed, producing the disease.

When it enters the body via the skin, a small red-brown pimple forms at the site of the infection. This gradually enlarges, blisters, hardens and then ulcerates, creating a crater with a black core.

As the infection spreads, the sufferer begins to feel extremely unwell. If it spreads into the bloodstream, the victim is likely to die.

When the bacterium is breathed in, it reproduces very quickly. A high fever and difficulty in breathing are followed by haemorrhage, as ulceration eats through the blood vessels. Shock, coma and death follow within hours.

Treatment
There is no question of home treatment for anthrax. All suspected cases have to be isolated and treated in hospital. The bacteria are killed by most antibiotics, but these only work in the early stages. The more serious lung infection is rarely responsive to treatment.

Prevention
The only way to prevent the disease among animals is by immunization. In cattle, any sudden death is treated as anthrax, unless disproven; the herd is destroyed and the carcases buried in quicklime.

Farm workers are always advised not to handle any dead animal unless it has been declared free of infection by the local veterinary inspector. Sheep can carry a skin infection caused by anthrax, so it is wise to keep away from animals with an obvious skin complaint.

A vaccine can be given to those at risk, and protective clothing and masks are essential for those who are disposing of infected materials.

Life cycle of an anthrax spore

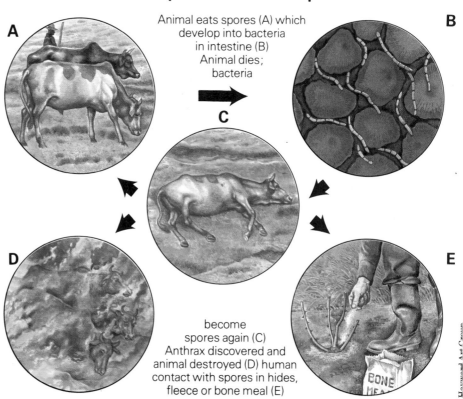

Animal eats spores (A) which develop into bacteria in intestine (B) Animal dies; bacteria become spores again (C) Anthrax discovered and animal destroyed (D) human contact with spores in hides, fleece or bone meal (E)

Antibiotics

Q Why doesn't my doctor prescribe an antibiotic when I get a sore throat, cold or cough?

A Because antibiotics are not likely to be effective against them. These drugs only work on diseases caused by bacteria. Colds, 'flu and most sore throats are carried by viruses, a different type of germ.

Q There are some old antibiotics in the medicine cupboard. Can I take them for the same problem as I took them for last year?

A No. Never take old antibiotics, or capsules prescribed for someone other than yourself. It could be dangerous. Always consult your doctor.

Q I am on the Pill. Will I have problems if I take an antibiotic?

A Most antibiotics do not affect the action of the contraceptive Pill, but one, called rifampicin, destroys the Pill in the body, making it ineffective. Another, ampicillin, makes the Pill less effective. So you should always remind the doctor that you are on the Pill.

Q Can I drink alcohol while I am on antibiotics?

A Most antibiotics have no ill-effects when combined with alcohol. Warnings about use with alcohol are almost always printed on the container in which the antibiotic is packed. In any event, your doctor will almost certainly advise you on this at the time he prescribes them for you.

Q Can antibiotics be taken during pregnancy?

A No drug should be taken during pregnancy unless it is essential for the mother's well-being. At present we have no certain way of testing whether drugs are safe for the unborn child. Although much animal testing is carried out, this does not give reliable information about human safety. Tetracyclines taken during pregnancy can cause discolouration in the teeth of a child. Your doctor will be well aware of the dangers and will advise you.

Antibiotics fight a great variety of infections and have conquered or controlled many widespread and deadly diseases. So how do these 'miracle drugs' work?

Being prescribed a course of antibiotics is such a common experience today that many people have forgotten that these drugs have made possible some of the most dramatic advances of modern medicine, and, of course, saved countless lives.

The first antibiotic, penicillin, was introduced in the 1940s. Since then the search for, and discovery of, new types has been almost continuous, and the various antibiotics have between them dramatically reduced the mortality rates from several of the world's severe diseases.

Life savers
Because of antibiotics, pneumonia is no longer a killer. The venereal diseases, syphilis and gonorrhoea, can be cured if detected early enough. People who catch typhoid usually need not fear for their lives. Sufferers from bronchitis, that persistent and distressing chest infection, can be helped considerably. Deaths from meningitis, an inflammation of the membranes which envelop the brain and spinal cord, are much fewer than they ever were.

Antibiotics are also used to combat infection in patients who have undergone surgery, or those with serious body wounds. Again, the number of lives saved is substantial.

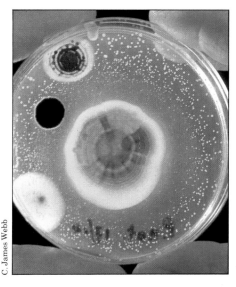

Above: Penicillin mould being cultured under laboratory conditions to produce an effective drug.
Right: Penicillin allergy rash.

And these drugs also cure many relatively minor problems such as throat infections, tonsillitis, cystitis (the urinary problem) abscesses, carbuncles, and septic fingers.

What they can do
Most of the time, we are exposed to what doctors and scientists call micro-organisms—in other words, germs. They are in food, in the air we breathe, in plants, the soil and in our own bodies. Most are harmless to human beings, many are beneficial, but a few are not and these cause disease.

Micro-organisms which cause disease are divided into a number of different types. Perhaps the three most commonly encountered are bacteria, viruses and protozoa. They all attack the body in different ways to cause different illnesses. Among the many conditions caused by bacteria are pneumonia and tuberculosis. Viruses cause such ailments as the common cold, flu, chicken pox, and smallpox. Protozoa bring about, among other things, amoebic dysentry and vaginal irritations.

Antibiotics are, quite simply, drugs which kill bacteria. They have no effect on viruses, are not prescribed for them, and, strictly speaking, are not used against protozoal infection either.

How they work
Antibiotics can be thought of as actually attacking micro-organisms, breaking them down and preventing their growth and multiplication within the body.

The most remarkable part of antibiotic action is that it is selective. This means that a given antibiotic drug only works on certain types of micro-organism, literally 'homing in' on the foreign bodies they are intended to kill, and leaving the other bacteria in the body unharmed.

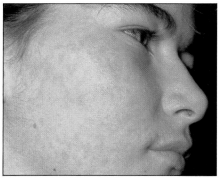

Antibiotics and their uses

Antibiotic	Uses
Penicillins The best-known, most widely used group. Common types: Penicillin G (usually injected), Penicillin V tables, Ampicillin capsules, Amoxicillin capsules and Talampicillin tablets	Some forms of tonsillitis, pneumonia, meningitis, syphilis, gonorrhoea, cystitis urinary infections, septic fingers, bronchitis, carbuncles
Tetracyclines A group of antibiotics developed after penicillin which considerably widened their effective range. Common types, usually taken by mouth, are Tetracycline itself, Oxytetracycline and a combination of the two	Infections of the respiratory (breathing) system; urinary infections; acne; rosacea (red nose); soft tissue infections such as some serious infections of the bones and sinuses
Erythromycin Common types, usually taken by mouth, are Erythrocin, Erythroped and Ilosone **Cotrimoxazole** Common types, taken as tablets, are Bactrium and Septrium	Respiratory infections; soft tissue infections Urinary infections and bronchitis Serious infections, especially of bones and sinuses
Cephalosporins The most recently developed group—originally discovered in a sewage effluent on the Mediterranean island of Sardinia. Chemical names include cephalexin and cephaloridine	Respiratory, genital, urinary, soft tissue and ear infections
Miscellaneous There is a large number of antibiotics of various types which are used more rarely. These include Chloromycetin, Streptomycin, Doxycycline, Gentamycin and Lincomycin	Each has a wide variety of types and may be effective in typhoid, meningitis and tuberculosis

Sulphonamides, which pre-date penicillin, are not actually antibiotics, but similar in action in that they fight bacteria and may be used against some infections for which antibiotics are also used. Some anti-protozoals, such as metronidazole (flagyl) are linked with antibiotics, but they are not, strictly speaking, the same.

To fully understand why antibiotics should be capable of this requires considerable specialist knowledge of chemistry. The basic theory, however, is fairly simple to understand. In nature, some micro-organisms just happen to attack and destroy others.

That this should be so was discovered by accident. The famous pathologist, Alexander Fleming, who discovered penicillin, noticed (as others had done before him without taking their findings any further) that certain bacteria stopped growing when placed close to the fungus called penicillium, most commonly found on mouldy bread.

The most active part of the penicillium fungus had then to be isolated to produce an effective antibiotic drug. With this knowledge of the chemical substances which kill micro-organisms, researchers could then move on to the next stage: copying them to produce artificial antibiotics. So now they are mostly produced artificially.

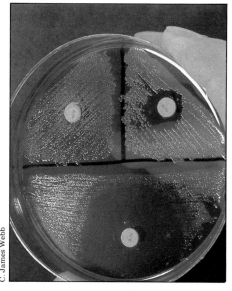

C. James Webb

Penicillin (centre each section) acting against different bacteria. Dark areas show strongest effects.

The fact that antibiotics occur naturally has meant that new ones have been discovered in what may seem to be extraordinary places. One, for example, was isolated from substances growing in dungheaps. But penicillin antibiotics remain to this day the most widely used.

Drawbacks
When antibiotics home in on bacteria, some will survive the attack, and, remarkable though it may seem, 'learn' from the experience how to resist similar action in future.

The more an antibiotic is used, the greater the number of bacteria learn to survive attack—in other words, build up 'resistance'.

So, in theory, antibiotics should be used as little as possible. If a bacteria becomes resistant to a certain antibiotic, as happened, for example, with the first penicillins, an alternative antibiotic has to be used. Luckily, the development of alternative and synthetic antibiotic types means that this is possible. This is one reason why researchers are continually developing new types.

Side-effects
Some people are allergic to penicillin, usually coming out in a rash when given it. They should always tell anyone who treats them medically if this is the case.

Many antibiotics can have side-effects, ranging from indigestion and diarrhoea to deafness and loss of balance. In most cases, it is a question of temporary discomfort to be tolerated for the sake of a permanent cure. However, you should always go back to your doctor without delay if an antibiotic is having a persistent, worrying side-effect.

Antibiotics really are 'miracle drugs', but like all precision instruments, they need to be used properly. Medically, this means tailoring the drug to the patient's infection. Bronchitis, or urinary problems may, for example, be caused by one bacteria in one attack, and a slightly different one the next. Each needs a particular antibiotic to treat it.

The side-effects of taking a wrong antibiotic can in some cases be very unpleasant, even dangerous. If you are being treated by a new doctor—especially abroad—tell him if you know of an antibiotic, or any other drug, that disagrees with you. Never take anyone else's antibiotics. Never take antibiotics given to you for a previous illness. Always complete a course of antibiotics given you: if you do not, the bacteria have a greater chance of 'learning' how to become immune, and the infection could get worse. Never take antibiotics without being supervised by a doctor.

Antiperspirant

Perspiration—or sweating—can be embarrassing, but today the wide range of antiperspirants on the market will help alleviate any excessive problem.

Q When I go to the chemist, I never know which type of antiperspirant to buy. Are some kinds better than others?

A Generally speaking, all the brands on offer are very similar in effect. However, the roll-on variety are slightly better because they cover the area more thoroughly. An aerosol spray quite often does not hit the mark so accurately and a lot of the antiperspirant can be lost when being applied. This makes them relatively expensive to use.

Q Whenever I use an antiperspirant, it seems to leave stains on my clothes. Why does this happen?

A This question raises several points. The first is that sweat itself can stain clothes quite badly, and no matter how good an antiperspirant you use, some will get through and leave its mark.

Then many of the clothes worn today can be very tight: jeans, T-shirts and so on. This encourages excessive sweating and the perspiration has less chance to evaporate, being in close contact with the fabric.

Finally, there is the antiperspirant itself. This contains a number of other substances apart from the active ingredients and these can rub off on clothes and leave stains. Some manufacturers try to reduce this problem by not using anything too oily. Unfortunately, these substances are very necessary to the product, as they help bind the salts to the skin so that they can be effective.

Q I am going to Greece for a holiday and am wondering whether I should use an antiperspirant there—or if it is better to allow the body to perspire freely?

A In countries which are very hot, it would be dangerous to prevent the body from sweating, but since antiperspirants are only used under the arms, there is little danger of this. The armpits contain a relatively small number of sweat glands compared with the body as a whole and so any reduction in their action will not seriously affect your body temperature.

Perspiring is a natural bodily function common to everyone. It can nevertheless be embarrassing to find that during hot weather or exercise we develop unpleasant smells and unsightly sweat stains on our clothes. For this reason, most of us rely on an antiperspirant to solve the problem of underarm perspiration.

Antiperspirants come in two forms, 'wet' (liquid) and 'dry' powder, and they are available as a roll-on, an atomizer spray or in aerosol cans. All these products are similar in effect if not in the way they control perspiration.

What is perspiration?

Perspiring—or sweating—is our main cooling mechanism. When the body gets too hot, it sends signals to the millions of sweat glands located all over its surface. These are activated to produce sweat—a watery, slightly salty liquid—which is secreted through the skin via the pores. Its function is to absorb heat and it evaporates during this process. The effect is to cool the blood vessels close to the surface of the skin, so enabling cool blood to be recirculated throughout the body.

Because armpits have a lot of body hair and are poorly ventilated, sweat tends to get trapped and cannot dry quickly. This provides a warm and fertile breeding ground for bacteria, which feed on the oil in the sweat, producing the odours that so

Of the two sweat glands—apocrine and eccrine—the apocrine is abundantly present in underarm and pubic areas. It is this gland antiperspirant especially acts on.

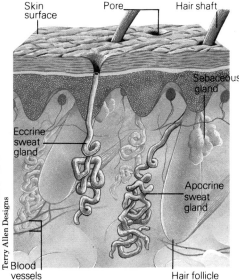

Skin surface — Pore — Hair shaft — Sebaceous gland — Eccrine sweat gland — Apocrine sweat gland — Blood vessels — Hair follicle

Terry Allen Designs

many people find offensive. Strict hygiene and scrupulous cleanliness can reduce this to a minimum in most cases.

How an antiperspirant works

A sweat gland resembles a tiny coiled tube. It opens on to the surface of the skin so that when a 'wet' antiperspirant is applied, the active ingredients it contains—aluminium salts—cause the gland to close up, and block the exit, preventing the escape of the sweat.

No-one seems to understand quite how the salts work, but certainly they are very effective. The sweat is prevented from reaching the air and is absorbed back into the body, simply and—as far as is known—harmlessly.

The 'dry' form of antiperspirant, of which talcum powder is a good example, works in a different way altogether. When the sweat reaches the surface of the skin, the antiperspirant soaks it up, and any smell is camouflaged.

Problems that can arise

Some people find that they are allergic to antiperspirants. If this happens, the simple remedy is to change to another brand. It is usually the additional substances in a particular make, such as the perfume, that cause the allergic reaction; the active antiperspirant ingredients seldom do, but when it does happen, it can lead to an unsightly and irritating skin rash. For this reason, antiperspirants should never be applied to broken skin, and warnings about this are printed on all bottles and cans.

Trouble can also occur if there is any lapse in general hygiene and applications of antiperspirant are not washed off before another is rolled or sprayed on. If the sweat ducts are blocked for too long, infection can arise, leading to boils.

Excessive perspiration

Some people find perspiration more of a problem than others. If it is so excessive that ordinary antiperspirants do not work, it might be worth a visit to the doctor who will try to identify the underlying cause and find a remedy. Otherwise, it is best to avoid all the things that cause more sweating than usual, such as getting too hot, eating and drinking too much or becoming over-excited or stressed. In very severe cases, the sweat glands under the arms can be removed, but this is very rarely done.

Anus

Q Is it true that eating curry makes the anus itch?

A Eating highly spiced food such as curry can provoke an irritation of the anus because of the spices in the faeces passing through the anal canal. If this is a problem, then avoidance of spicy food is the best cure.

Q The last couple of times that I have been to the toilet, I have noticed blood on the toilet paper. Could this be serious?

A It is always wise to consult your doctor if you notice blood in your faeces or on the toilet paper or experience any bleeding from the anus. The underlying problem, when finally diagnosed, may well be a minor one, but it is not worth taking any risks.

Q My baby has diarrhoea and a rash has developed round his anus. What should I do?

A Diarrhoea can cause a rash to develop in the anal area due to continual irritation. To clear it up quickly, change the baby's nappies as soon as they become dirty and clean the affected area thoroughly with mild soap and water. Then dress the area with soothing antiseptic cream or zinc ointment. Fresh air is also an effective healer, so it is a good idea to allow your baby to play for a while without a nappy on.

Q I am sometimes woken up in the night by an intense pain in my anus and back passage, but it seems to have nothing to do with passing faeces. What is the cause, and should I see a doctor?

A The type of fleeting pain has the odd-sounding medical name of proctalgia fugax and is thought to be caused by spasms of the muscles in the lower part of the alimentary canal. It appears to be brought on by anxiety. The best way to deal with the pain is to get up and have a glass of water, or a hot drink. The pain should gradually subside. If it persists, occurs frequently or is adding to your worries, then by all means you should discuss the matter with your doctor.

Once all the goodness has been extracted from the food we eat, the unwanted residue is excreted via the anus. But this is a sensitive area where irritating or painful disorders can occur; fortunately, these usually respond well to treatment.

The anus or anal canal is the very last section of the digestive system. It is about 10 cm (4in) long and is the opening through which the body's solid waste products—known as faeces—are excreted.

How it works

As the faeces near the end of their journey down the intestines, they gradually harden as liquids are absorbed by the body and the solid waste is pushed into the rectum. At the end of the anus are two rings of muscle, known as the internal and external sphincters. Normally the two spincters keep the anus closed, but during defaecation—the passing of faeces—they relax to allow it to escape. The internal sphincter (which is under the control of the nervous system) senses the presence of the faeces and relaxes, allowing them to enter the anal canal. The external sphincter is kept closed deliberately (a skill we learn in babyhood) until a convenient moment presents itself when the faeces can be passed. To ease the passage of the faeces from the anus, the tissue in the lining of the canal secretes a lubricating fluid called mucus.

Anal problems

Problems in the anus range from the wildly irritating to the extremely uncomfortable, and most people will at some time or other suffer from an anal irritation of some sort. However, anal problems are most common in childhood, pregnancy and from middle age onwards. To help prevent some of them, it is sensible to wash the area regularly with warm water and mild unscented soap; dry with a soft towel.

Difficulty in the passing of hard faeces often results in other trouble. The lining of the anal canal is quite delicate and passing hard motions can tear the lining. Not only does this mean that infection can enter the wound—known as an anal fissure—but it can become extremely painful to defaecate. Unfortunately, the problem is often difficult to deal with as the sufferer may try to hold back the faeces to avoid the pain. This has the effect of hardening the faeces even further and so worsening the situation. Usually the problem is treated with antibiotics for the infection and a laxative to soften the faeces.

In the long term, the best way to prevent this problem, which can affect both adults and children, is to eat a diet rich in bran and roughage. This has the effect of speeding the passage of faeces through the last part of the alimentary canal and makes the faeces softer because there is less time available for water to be absorbed back into the blood vessels

The small pattern of cracks in this anus are called fissures and are usually caused by passing a hard or very large, awkward stool. Because of constantly repeated irritation (further motions), fissures do not heal easily.

The development of a boil in the anus can lead to a fistula. The boil bursts but does not usually drain into the anus. Instead, drainage channels form through the skin and open to the outside of the body beside the anus.

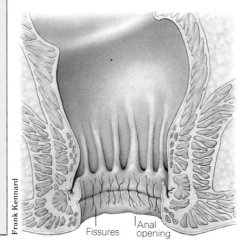

Fissures | Anal opening

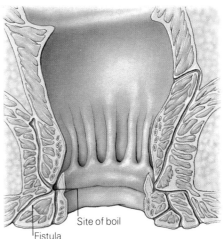

Site of boil | Fistula

Frank Kennard

Common causes of pain in the anal area

Symptoms	Possible cause	Action
Sharp pain during bowel movement and pain or aching for up to an hour afterwards; bleeding from anus	Anal fissure	Apply soothing ointment; have a warm salt bath for temporary relief; see a doctor. A lubricant may be prescribed and surgery recommended to remove the affected tissue and stretch the anal opening
Soreness not made better or worse by defaecation; discharge from anal region	Anal fistula	See a doctor. Antibiotics will be prescribed; an operation may be needed
Severe, throbbing pain	Abscess or boil	See a doctor. The pus will need to be surgically drained
Intense pain, not worse on passing faeces; anus painful to touch, may itch; painful deep purple protrusion may appear on one side of anus	External piles	Apply ice cold water on a tissue or have a hot bath for temporary relief; see a doctor. Long term, take more exercise; eat more roughage; surgery may be needed
No pain but itching, soreness and the passage of much mucus; bright red blood may be lost on defaecation; feeling of fullness in anus	Internal piles	See a doctor. An injection will provide temporary relief but surgical treatment will probably be needed
Pain may be worse on defaecation; protrusion of pink tissue from anus	Prolapse (dropping) of rectum	See a doctor. An operation will probably be necessary, but in the case of a child the doctor may be able to push the collapsed part back into place

lining the canal. And a high roughage diet is helpful in preventing other anal problems such as piles and some disorders of the large intestine.

Further disorders
The most well-known of anal problems is piles (haemorrhoids). These are caused by abnormalities of the blood vessels surrounding the anal canal, forming clumps of swollen, contorted varicose veins both inside and outside the anus. According to their position piles are thus known as internal or external. They are extremely

In a prolapse, the muscles surrounding the rectum become weakened so that during defaecation part of the rectum collapses and protrudes from the anus. To solve this problem the rectum may need stitching back into place.

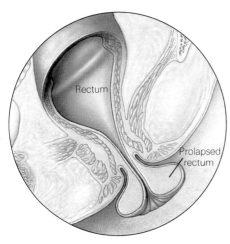
Rectum
Prolapsed rectum

uncomfortable, cause irritation and itching, and are often accompanied by bleeding. Happily, if suppositories fail the piles can now be treated with injections or by surgery, if the condition is severe.

In children
Children are often susceptible to irritations around the anal opening and in younger children this is usually caused by nappy rash. Another anal irritation which is more common in children than adults is caused by threadworms—a type of parasite that lives in the lower bowel—and these cause severe itching around the anus, but can be treated with drugs.

In adults
In adulthood, constant itching of the anus—known as pruritius ani—can be caused by infection of the skin around the anus or by severe anxiety. Scratching the area can result in considerable skin damage, causing the infection to spread and the area to bleed.

The best treatments are antiseptic ointments to kill the bacteria and calamine lotion to cool the inflammation. But a doctor should be consulted as itching and irritation can be associated with other anal problems. In any disease of the spinal cord the sphincteral muscles may be paralyzed, resulting in an inability to control excretion.

Boils and abscesses are the most common types of infection in the anal canal, and they can be very uncomfortable—abscesses particularly so. This is

because a bad abscess can form a drainage channel—called a fistula—that opens to the outside of the body next to the anus. The fistula takes the form of a small red spot from which fluid leaks. This complaint is normally treated with antibiotics, and, in severe cases, surgery.

Complications
A further complication can also arise through the weakening of the internal muscles that surround the rectum. This leads to the lining of the rectum dropping, a complaint called a prolapse. It is easily indentifiable as the lining can be seen protruding from the anal opening. The weakness may be present at birth or develop with old age, or it can be brought on by pushing too hard during defaecation, by diarrhoea, whooping cough or during labour. The complaint should always be reported to the doctor who will either push the lining back into position or, if the problem is severe, he or she may find it necessary to secure the lining with a few stitches.

Unwanted growths may also protrude from the anus. These normally take the form of benign lumps of tissue called polyps and they are particularly common in young children. Warts and wart-like tumours called papillomata may also occur, especially in middle and old age. In both cases the doctor may recommend diathermy, in which the growths are burned off electrically. However, the presence of papillomata necessitates surgical removal because they can lead to cancer.

Anxiety

Q **What is the most important thing I can do when I have an attack of anxiety?**

A One of the most helpful things you can do is stop, take some deep breaths, relax and think about what is causing your attack. One of the commonest problems with anxiety is panic, so that a sufferer is not able to deal with his or her anxiety calmly.

Q **Can I die of anxiety?**

A In real life one doesn't die of anxiety, but it is possible to die of side-effects, such as a heart attack brought on by an anxiety-producing situation. But anxiety is a relatively minor problem and you should be able to cope with it fairly easily.

Q **What if my doctor prescribes drugs such as tranquillizers or sleeping pills? Can I become addicted to them?**

A Unfortunately yes, particularly the sleeping pills. It's all too easy to use drugs to become calm and, seemingly, to remove the symptoms and even the causes of anxiety. But they are really only useful for helping you to alter your behaviour pattern or re-learn how to cope with the things that cause your anxiety. But this can be done without drugs—by seeking professional help and through sheer willpower.

Q **Am I the only person who suffers from anxiety?**

A No, certainly not. Almost everyone suffers from anxiety at some time in their lives. This can be something as simple as an anxiety based on superstition, like fear of the number 13. There are organizations set up to help all forms of anxiety. Your doctor should have a list.

Q **Can babies feel anxiety?**

A Yes, frequently. Being hungry or left alone can be terrifying for an infant who cannot communicate verbally. Only the repeated experience of being comforted and cared for will create a feeling of trust and reduce anxiety.

It is perfectly normal to feel anxious from time to time, but intense anxiety which disrupts the sufferer's life needs professional treatment.

We have all felt anxious at some time, whether we call it feeling uneasy, on edge or uptight. It is perfectly natural to feel anxious and, in fact, to some degree it can have good effects such as toning us up for a big match or sharpening awareness for an interview or exam.

But some forms of anxiety are not as healthy as others. If you get mildly worked up before an exam, that can be beneficial. However, if you cannot sleep well the night before, or begin to sweat profusely and feel nauseated as you enter the examination hall, this is a more serious anxiety attack and if you find that this is part of a continuing pattern, you should seek help.

A child's anxiety is readily dispelled by the loving reassurance of his mother.

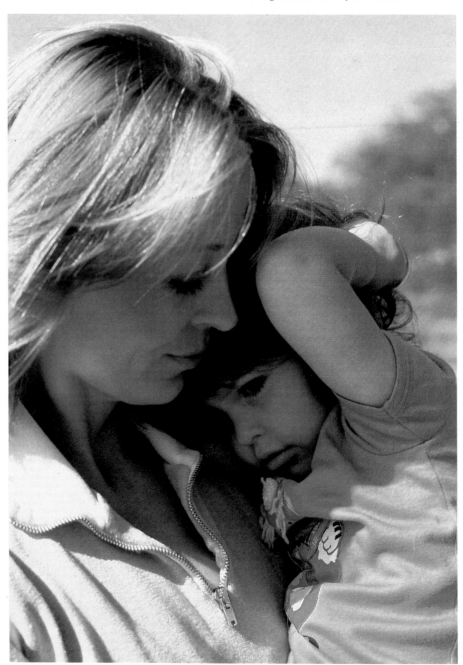

What is anxiety?

Our reaction to stress is an inbuilt survival mechanism that originally enabled us to act instantly when our lives were threatened. To prepare for action the heartbeat strengthens to pump blood to all the muscles, and blood pressure rises. Because the muscles need fuel to produce energy, blood sugar is released into the bloodstream and the oxygen required to turn this sugar into energy is taken into the lungs with quickened breathing, even gasping. Because the body has a limited supply of blood, some has to be diverted from other systems, so the blood supply to the stomach is reduced and digestion is disturbed. The mouth goes dry, the pupils dilate and, as the body overheats with increased blood supply to the muscles, the skin begins to sweat to cool it down. Adrenalin is released from the adrenal glands and keeps the stress reactions going.

When action has been taken and the danger is over or the problem resolved, the body relaxes and returns to normal once more. But when the threat is low-level and continuous as is common in the emotionally stressful situations of modern living, often no direct action can be taken to deal with it and the body will suffer the effects of long-term tension.

This is what is happening to the anxious person lying awake at 3 a.m. with a pounding heart and a stomach tied in knots over a purely emotional problem at work, for example. He is suffering from the same physical and chemical changes that were originally intended to save life, only now the reactions are inappropriate to the events.

Anxiety takes many forms. Some have obvious causes, as a fear of dogs in someone who was bitten or frightened by one as a child. Other forms are not so clear and may include anxiety about a relationship which can make you sexually impotent or frigid. Sometimes the cause of anxiety can be totally imaginary—a groundless fear that you are in line for the sack, for instance. Occasionally the anxiety takes an unspecific form, such as sudden, unexplained panic on the way to the office or a sense of general hopelessness about the state of the world (called 'angst').

Anxiety sufferers

Anxiety is experienced by both men and women, though women tend to seek help for it more than men. What is interesting is that there appear to be several times in life when people are more likely to suffer from anxiety.

The first of these times is the period of adolescence when young people are coming to terms with their own identi-

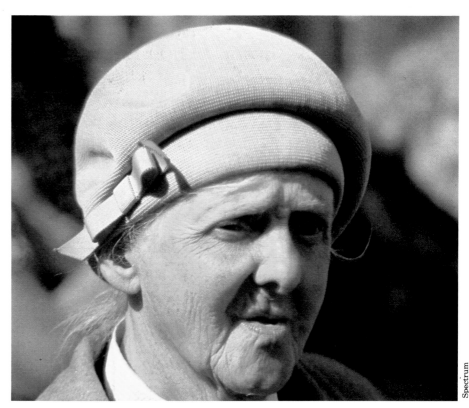

ties. Many of their anxieties are of a sexual nature or are an expression of the teenager's self-doubts.

This is aggravated by the need to be accepted by society based on its values— good looks, brightness, likeability—and also by the competitiveness among young people.

In the early thirties there is a new peak of anxiety. People begin to worry about success in their jobs and their incomes being sufficient for their needs. Men especially are concerned about whether or not they 'are going to make it to the top'. Marital conflicts, or potential ones, that could have been ignored or put aside in earlier years may come to the surface only now.

During their late forties or early fifties men and women tend to look back and perhaps feel a certain disappointment that they have not done better, or panic because there seems to be so little time left and so much still to accomplish. Because of hormonal changes at this time of life (part of the menopause, or 'change of life' when periods cease and the ability to bear children ends), women are especially vulnerable.

The later years of life can also bring new anxiety for both men and women. This is often related to loneliness and the feeling on the part of the older person that he or she is isolated from everyone else.

Dealing with physical and emotional 'growing pains' can be a source of anxiety.

Tension in the elderly many be caused by feelings of being isolated from others.

Causes

There are two main theories about the causes of anxiety. The first holds that it is due to a personality disorder that makes our psychological defences unable to work in the way they should. In other words, instead of recognizing the anxiety

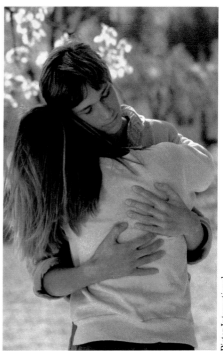

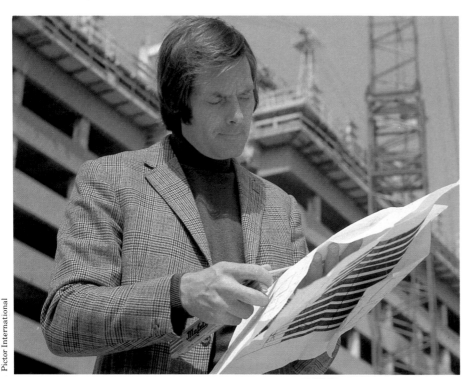

Pictor International

symptoms and dealing with them, the sufferer turns the symptoms into a pattern—one that is often self-destructive.

The second theory claims that there is a failure in some physical function, especially in the nervous system. This may be due to an imbalance of chemicals in the body. Supporters of this theory believe that these 'malfunctions' can be cured by effective and painless drug therapy.

Thirdly, some theorists suggest that the causes of the problem are much simpler than either of these theories suggest and that anxiety, in fact, is merely a result of modern life: the widespread loss of social and religious values and a response to conditions over which we no longer feel we have any control.

Symptoms

It can be said that anxiety is increased arousal about a particular event and that some people may become over-aroused when the specific trigger for their anxiety occurs, like a deadline that must be met. They then become over-excited and develop the physical symptoms associated with coping with an external threat: increased heartbeat, high blood pressure, excessive sweating, and rapid breathing resulting sometimes in giddiness or weakness at the knees.

Prolonged contraction of the muscles, readied for action, may cause cramp-like spasm, backache, the tender, aching spots in shoulders and neck so familiar to tense people, or headaches brought on by tensed forehead muscles or continually gritting the teeth. Digestive disorders

In their thirties people are prone to worry about success in their careers.

may include spastic colon, indigestion, nausea, stomach cramps, and gastric ulcers. And because the digestive and urinary systems are 'working overtime', this may cause an endless number of visits to the toilet.

Other common symptoms are insomnia, chest pain, asthma, sexual difficulties, a lump in the throat or an inability to swallow, and migraine headaches, possibly precipitated by biochemical and physical changes in the body.

If the anxiety continues, secondary symptoms can develop; these can include skin rashes, spots, weight problems (under- or overweight). Strangely enough, those suffering from anxiety can also experience either increased aggression or the reverse effect, becoming completely inhibited, withdrawn and even extremely depressed.

The symptoms are unpredictable and the effects can be disruptive in everyday life. Though anxiety can occur at any time, attacks are more likely to be associated with a specific situation, like dealing with a marital problem, fear of the boss, learning a particular subject at school.

If the symptoms are bad, there will be a certain amount of discomfort, both physical and social—people are often not very understanding when others are suf-

Even a mild case of anxiety reveals itself in facial expressions and gestures.

fering from anxiety. But the worst effects are that some of the symptoms are physically weakening (such as inability to sleep which causes further complications like irritability) and, if they are bad, may prevent you participating fully in certain aspects of your life, as for example when spots or a rash occurs before an important event.

Treatment

It is possible to try and cope with anxiety on your own. The first thing to do is to recognize and accept the symptoms and try to discover and face the causes.

But, if this self-help process is not enough—even with the aid of family and friends—it is best for you to consult the doctor. He or she may refer you to a psychotherapist who will help you discover and cope with the causes. This treatment may be carried out either in individual sessions or in the company of other anxiety sufferers in group psychotherapy.

Many doctors are suggesting alternative therapies, the purpose of most of them being to help you relax and gain a greater self-awareness. These may include yoga, breathing exercises, biofeedback or even meditation.

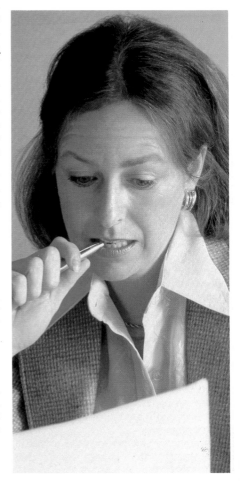

Self-help with anxiety

Though it might seem unthinkable when you are in the grip of anxiety, there are positive steps you can take to overcome your symptoms.

● The first and most important step is to accept and come to terms with the fact that you are under stress. Anxiety is nothing to be ashamed of, so don't try to deny that you are prey to the same stresses that everyone else is or to assume that they are coping marvellously while you are a bundle of nerves. Anxiety-related illnesses are among the most common, and a good many of the people you meet everyday are probably suffering from some of the same symptoms as you.

● Recognize your symptoms for what they are so as to reduce their emotional charge. Worrying about the dizziness, the tightness in your chest, the lump in your throat or whatever can send you spiralling into a panic and make you even less able to cope. You may need practical help from your doctor for a while.

● Try to find out what is at the root of your anxiety. What are you afraid of? Is there some conflict involved? If your anxiety is due to your general life style, you should think carefully about what you are doing and why it is harming you.

● Many women feel more anxious around their periods because the hormone imbalance affects their emotions. If you think this might be true for you, make a chart of your menstrual cycle for two or three months. In addition to marking the days on which you have your periods, make a record of the days on which you are emotionally upset. Study the chart to see if a pattern emerges. If it does, it is likely that your stress reactions are associated with your menstrual cycles, so plan your life accordingly. Use your good days to the full, and on your low days plan to take life more easily and try to relax.

● If your anxiety is making it practically impossible to cope even with the smallest tasks, try breaking them down into manageable units and set yourself very modest goals, doing more as you gain confidence. Don't put off unpleasant or threatening tasks.

● Keep active. Even if you feel shattered, don't admit defeat and go to bed or flop in front of the television. Instead, take up an engrossing hobby like needlework or some other absorbing pastime that will fully engage your mind and keep it from gnawing away at itself. This will refresh you more than nervous inactivity (unless you add to your anxiety by being a perfectionist).

● Keep regular habits. A set routine can give you a firm foundation even if the rest of your day seems chaotic. Eat balanced meals, go to bed at a reasonable hour (even if you can't sleep), and in the morning get up and dressed even if you're not going out. Take care over your appearance.

● Avoid coffee and cigarettes as far as possible because they increase stress. And the dangers of using alcohol to combat anxiety need hardly be emphasized, especially if your doctor has already given you medication to help.

● Incorporate both relaxation and exercise into your daily routine. Relaxation techniques like yoga and breathing exercises can help calm you down and overcome the fatigue caused by tense muscles. And strenuous exercise like sports or even running up the stairs will use up some of the energy the body produces as a reaction to stress. If this kind of activity is not possible at a given, stressful moment, use the 'Stop' emergency technique. Say 'Stop' sharply to yourself, then breathe in and, as you breathe out, slowly relax your hands and arms. Then breathe in again and, as you breathe out, relax your jaw—you will probably find that your teeth were tightly clenched. Let your jaw drop completely and then breathe calmly once or twice before you go on with what you were doing, but take it easy.

● Avoid bottling up your emotions, though if you need to let off some steam, don't take your feelings out on an innocent party. Instead try bashing a pillow until you are exhausted.

● Finally, talk your problems over with someone sympathetic who can help put them in perspective and provide moral support. You'll find a happy family life can give you a tremendous boost, and turning your attention to others has the added effect of taking your mind off your own troubles.

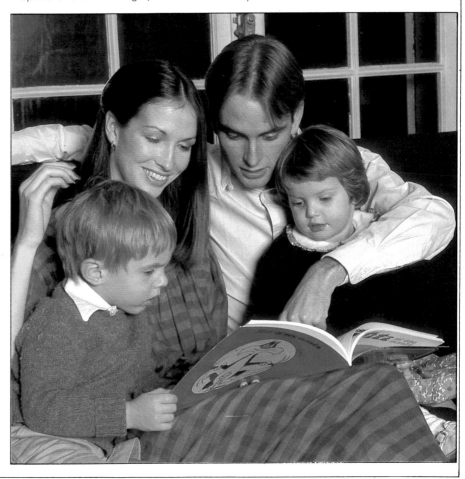

A rich, warm family relationship is a good foundation for security which is a safeguard against anxiety.

Aphasia

Aphasia is the loss of the ability to understand words and communicate through speech. It can be caused by injury or disease, but speech therapy can encourage recovery.

There are two important processes in the brain which control the power of speech. First, when a spoken message is received by the brain via the ears, the person is normally able to follow what is being said because the brain uses the memory to decode the sounds. Then, secondly, an answer is prepared. Ideas are turned into words (encoded), again using the memory to co-ordinate the process, and the muscles of the larynx (throat), jaw, lips and tongue are stimulated by the brain, enabling the person to speak and give the answer. These two processes take place in areas of the brain linked by nerves.

Receiving and decoding the spoken (and written) word takes place in the upper part of the right lobe of the human brain. When things go wrong here, the term used is sensory or receptive aphasia. Encoding the spoken word takes place in the left lobe of the brain, and upset or disturbance here is called motor or expressive aphasia.

Causes in adults

A range of diseases and conditions can produce adult aphasia, but the commonest of these are complaints which affect the flow of arterial blood to the speech centres of the brain. These include cerebral artery thrombosis (clotting), cerebral artery haemorrhage and cerebral artery embolism (a foreign clot lodging in the blood vessels). They produce weakness in the limbs on the right side of the body or paralysis (a 'stroke') and the aphasia accompanies the power loss.

Head injuries which result from domestic, road or works accidents or violent assault can also damage the centres of speech causing sensory or motor aphasia, or both together.

Rarer conditions affecting the brain such as cerebral tumours, cerebral degeneration and damage following infection of the brain may sometimes produce forms of aphasia.

How the brain enables us to communicate

Words are heard (A); sound is received by primary auditory cortex (B), deciphered in Wernicke's area (C) and transmitted by nerves—arcuate fasciculus—(D) to Broca's area (E) where reply is formed and message sent to face via motor cortex (F), which also stimulates muscles of lips, tongue, jaw and throat to produce speech.

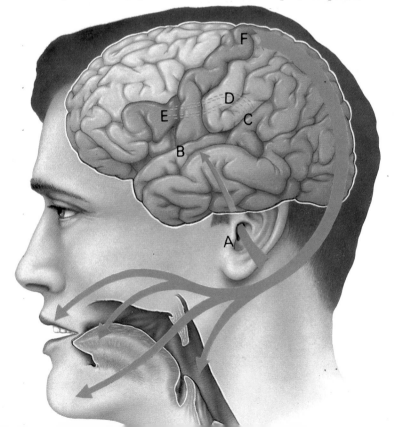

Types of adult aphasia

In the most severe form of adult motor or expressive aphasia, the individual may be left with only one or two words of expression, such as 'yes' or 'no', and even these may be used inappropriately. If there is no sensory or receptive aphasia, however, the motor aphasic person can still follow and understand speech and can carry out instructions.

This is important where the 'stroke' patient, for example, is being re-taught to use weak or paralyzed muscles and to carry out activities of daily living which restore his independence.

Severe motor aphasia is extremely frustrating for the sufferer since he or she cannot communicate thoughts and needs quickly and accurately. Writing, which is a form of motor language is unfortunately similarly affected.

In less severe forms, the person has more vocabulary, but it is still much less than he had before he became ill. He may tend to repeat fixed words or phrases in a stereotyped fashion, a form of aphasia called *palilalia*. His speech generally is hesitant and may be filled with more gaps than usual.

The least severe but still frustrating form of motor aphasia is *nominal* or amnestic aphasia. In this condition, the individual recognizes familiar objects but is unable to give them the appropriate

In treating an aphasic child, the speech therapist will first establish how much, if any, language the child already has and will then help to develop this.

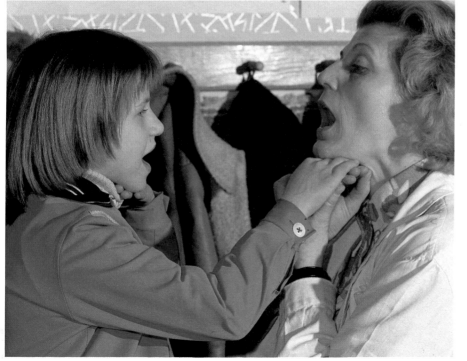

names. For example, the person can demonstrate that a pen is an object to write with but cannot state directly that this is 'a pen'.

Another feature of some motor aphasic sufferers is that, although their ordinary vocabulary may be limited to a few words, they can still swear. There is no known medical reason for this.

Although the power to understand and follow the spoken word is limited or grossly disturbed in sensory or receptive aphasia, the person may speak quite fluently and noisily. The difficulty is that what is said may not make any sense to the listener because grammer and sound may be quite distorted, yet the speaker is unaware of this. This form of sensory aphasia is sometimes called *jargon* aphasia. Where the same nonsense phases are constantly repeated, this is described as *echolalia*.

Aphasia in children

Speech is a complex skill which children have to learn. For the skill to be mastered, the child's brain must function properly and the two speech centres must be intact. The child must be exposed to sounds and words, and must have the full articulation equipment, that is, the muscles of the jaw, face and larynx must co-ordinate properly.

Aphasia in children is therefore essentially a problem of speech learning and it can be caused by a range of handicaps, one or several of which may occur together. These include brain damage which may have happened before

or during birth, spastic weakness, partial deafness, subnormal intelligence, and the condition known as autism (an emotional disorder in which the child completely withdraws from the real world, and is almost unable to communicate).

As well as showing symptoms of aphasia affecting adults, children also show other disturbances in their difficulties with words as symbols. There may be a failure to match the written and the spoken word. The child may try to read from right to left in a language normally read from left to right. Spelling words aloud or in spelling tests may reveal word difficulties. Parts of words may be moved around, creating bizarre results. Associated disturbances include the reading problem of dyslexia, or word blindness, and the writing problem of dysgraphia, or inability to form words.

Mothers generally notice speech delay and if this is pointed out to the family doctor or nursery school teacher, the child can be referred to a neurologist and an educational psychologist who can advise on possible improvement and recommend speech therapy or other training.

Treatment

The treatment of all forms of aphasia is nowadays undertaken by a qualified speech therapist, who works alongside the medical, nursing and physiotherapy staff where they are nursing a patient with a stroke or head injury.

To restore communication with the adult motor aphasic patient the therapist uses picture cards showing various common needs like food, toilet, washing or drinking, to which the patient can point. Alphabet cards and sheets may then be used which the patient can point to and use to construct words to get his message across. Stroke patients may be taught to write using the unaffected hand. Crosswords—spoken aloud—and tapes are also used as aids to speech recovery.

Strangely enough, the motor aphasic patient may sing quite fluently, even though speech is disturbed, and this can be used to communicate.

Family, friends and relatives can be helpful in talking to and encouraging the speech of the motor aphasic patient. Because of the patient's lack of ability to understand the treatment of severe sensory or receptive aphasia is difficult, but patients can sometimes be helped by the constant repetition of simple activities.

With motor aphasic children the aim is to teach speech instead of capitalize on speech existing before illness. The speech therapist first does a 'language search' to find out how much language the young child has, then tries to enlarge this.

Appendicitis

Q I am a model for a swimwear firm and have to have my appendix out. Will I have an ugly scar afterwards?

A This rarely happens today. Various ways of sealing wounds have been devised which improve the cosmetic appearance of an operation scar. In any case, the scar from your appendix operation will be below the 'bikini line' so your job should not be affected.

Q Do people always pass wind after an appendix operation? I would be so embarrassed if this happened to me.

A Far from being an embarrassment, wind is a sign that the bowels are returning to life. After any abdominal operation, the bowels stop working for a while. In fact, food and drink cannot be taken until 'bowel sounds' return. The bowels are full of wind anyway, and as they gain strength, this is the first thing to be expelled.

Q My brother, who is a sailor, has a grumbling appendix. What would happen if it suddenly worsened while he was at sea?

A Obviously, if away from medical help, some treatment has to be tried, whether at sea or on a mountain top. Painkillers are essential and antibiotics may help. A large vessel may have a ship's doctor who is well qualified to deal with such an emergency; otherwise, modern communications are so rapid that air-sea rescue services can be called in to cope with any crisis that may occur.

Q I am planning a world trip and will undoubtedly visit places with no medical facilities. Since I have had attacks of appendicitis in the past, is it possible to have my appendix removed as a preventative measure?

A This is sometimes done, but not as a general rule. In the 'developed world' the dangers of an unnecessary operation may outweigh the risks of sudden appendicitis. But in your case it may be a sensible precaution. Your doctor will be able to advise you.

The appendix is a small organ that was useful to our ancestors but is now virtually redundant. However, it can still cause trouble and sometimes has to be removed, but with modern surgical techniques, an appendectomy is both speedy and safe.

The appendix is a narrow, tube-like piece of gut resembling a tail, which is located at the end of the large intestine. The tip of the tube is closed; the other end joins on to the large intestine. It can be up to 10 cm (4 in) long and about 1.5 cm (5/8 in) in diameter.

It is only found in humans, certain species of apes and in the wombat. Other animals have an organ in the same position as the appendix that acts as an additional stomach, where cellulose, the fibrous part of plants, is digested by bacteria. It seems that as we evolved through the ages and began to eat less cellulose in favour of more meat, a special organ was no longer needed for its digestion. The appendix could therefore be described as a relic of evolution.

Appendicitis

Facts about the appendix appear to contradict one another. On the one hand, nature appears to have adapted it to act as a watchdog for infection at the lower end of the gut. Like the tonsils and adenoids, it contains a large collection of lymph glands for this purpose; but if the appendix does become inflamed, a condition called appendicitis results and the organ may have to be removed. On the other hand, the appendix seems by no means essential to health. It can be dispensed with at an early age, making no apparent difference, and has nearly shrivelled up completely by the age of 40 or so.

Appendicitis can occur at any time, from babyhood to old age. However, it is rare under the age of two, more common among teenagers, and then becomes increasingly rare again over the age of 30. Why it should reach its peak in youth remains a mystery.

Causes

In fact, the history and incidence of the condition is extremely baffling. Up to the end of the 19th century, it was relatively unknown. This is still so in places like Asia, Africa and Polynesia. But in Europe, North America and Australia, for example, appendicitis is now a very common complaint.

The reason for this is thought to be directly related to changes in our eating

An inflamed appendix and its position in the body

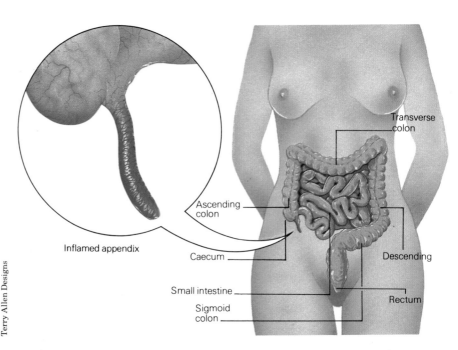

Inflamed appendix

Transverse colon

Ascending colon

Caecum

Small intestine

Sigmoid colon

Descending

Rectum

Terry Allen Designs

habits. The modern western diet has become so refined that it now lacks sufficient fibre—called roughage. This deficiency causes the food to slow down in its passage through the intestines. This sluggishness can lead to blockages, which may be a cause of appendicitis. Food residues can occasionally collect in the appendix and form an obstruction. Pips, fruit stones and other foreign bodies that may have been swallowed accidentally can also aggravate the appendix, but these are fortunately among the rarer causes of appendicitis.

Worms, the result of eating contaminated food, are another danger to the appendix. These intestinal parasites may lodge there and eventually cause an obstruction. Whatever their origin, blockages of any kind can lead to the onset of appendicitis.

The 'grumbling' appendix
Recurrent attacks of appendicitis, each lasting a day or two, can sometimes occur. As the appendix gets inflamed, the intestines nearby close round it to wall off the infection. If the inflammation clears up, the intestines may still be left stuck around the appendix. These 'adhesions' can restrain the normal movement of food around the system, resulting in colicky (griping) pains, which may then be felt in the appendix region during normal digestion. This gives rise to a 'grumbling' appendix, which will settle if it does not become inflamed again.

Serious symptoms
For various reasons, a bout of appendicitis may not clear up on its own: the appendix is blocked and further action will be necessary.

The early symptoms of appendicitis are not easy to distinguish from any other form of tummyache. Pain, which comes and goes in a colicky fashion is felt around the umbilicus (tummy button), as the appendix muscles contract while trying to drive any obstruction out. If there is no obstruction, then there will just be a constant ache.

After six to 12 hours, the symptoms will change, as inflammation builds up around the appendix. The overlying peritoneum (lining) of the abdomen becomes irritated and, as this is well supplied with nerves, more pain is felt around the appendix. Usually, this is in the right lower abdomen. However, the site of the maximum pain is variable.

Diagnosis
Often the patient has to press his or her own stomach to establish where it hurts most. The most common site is two-thirds of the way along a line joining the top of

Recognizing appendicitis

Early symptoms	Action
Colicky (griping) pain in stomach that comes and goes	Give mild painkiller e.g. paracetamol
Loss of appetite	Try a soothing drink: warm milk or weak tea
Constipation	Give a hot water bottle
	DO NOT GIVE A LAXATIVE—this will be harmful, causing painful contractions of the appendix and increasing the chance of perforation
In children, a respiratory infection may show symptoms imitating appendicitis. These *could* be genuine	TELL THE DOCTOR ABOUT TUMMY SYMPTOMS IN CHILD—just in case

Later symptoms Give no more home remedies. GET MEDICAL HELP AT ONCE

More pain in appendix area (right lower abdomen)	Patient lies with right leg flexed up. Stretching it down produces pain.
Pain may move up or down from umbilicus (tummy button)	Diarrhoea possible, but constipation more common
Slight rise in temperature e.g. 37.5°C (99.5°F)	Nausea
Slight increase in pulse rate	Vomiting
	Foul-smelling breath

Means of viewing the appendix

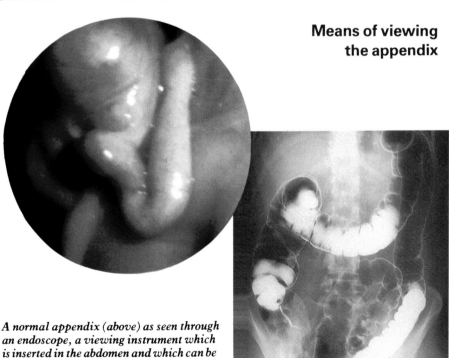

A normal appendix (above) as seen through an endoscope, a viewing instrument which is inserted in the abdomen and which can be used to take photographs inside the body. This is how a healthy appendix appears (right) when X-rayed.

Vision International

Q A great-aunt of mine died of appendicitis. Could this happen nowadays?

A This is most unlikely. In the past, any operation was fraught with dangers. As a result, an appendix operation was often delayed until perforation occurred and the patient would then become rapidly ill and even die.

Q Several members of my family have had to have their appendix out. Is this just a coincidence or can a tendency to appendicitis be inherited?

A Yes, it is possible that you have an inherited tendency. It may be that you have all inherited a similarly shaped appendix. One that is long and thin will block more easily than one that is short and stubby, and so cause appendicitis.

Q I am 45 and have heard that it is highly unlikely that I will ever have appendicitis at my age. Is this true?

A Yes, it is. If you have reached middle life without having had appendicitis, the chances are that you are unlikely to get it now because the appendix shrivels as you get older and is completely shrivelled by the age of 45—so it is not likely to become irritated and inflamed. This is why appendicitis tends to be a complaint of young people.

Q I have heard that swallowing cherry stones can lead to appendicitis. As they are my favourite fruit, I am worried that I may get this problem. Is there any truth in this?

A When appendectomies were first performed years ago, surgeons thought that the small hard lumps they found in the appendix were cherry stones because they looked like them, but in fact they were fecoliths—that is, small lumps of faeces which had become trapped in the appendix because it leads nowhere. So you can continue eating your favourite fruit because swallowing fruit stones usually results in their being excreted from the body in the normal way and only very rarely will they cause any irritation to the appendix.

the umbilicus to the top of the pelvic bone. This is called McBurney's point, after the American surgeon who first noted it. But the pain can move to the upper abdomen or down in the pelvis. In a woman, this is particularly confusing as it can be mimicked by gynaecological pains from the ovaries or womb. A rectal examination by the doctor may be needed to establish whether this pain is, in fact, caused by an inflamed, tender appendix.

The inflamed appendix often lies on the right leg muscle where it joins the back. Because this makes the leg stiff, the patient naturally bends the leg up to gain relief. Stretching it down then produces pain. The muscles in the front wall of the abdomen also go into spasm to protect the appendix from any painful movements the patient may make.

It may also be difficult, initially, for the doctor to diagnose appendicitis in children. The child may have a chest infection, with symptoms that imitate appendicitis, which disappear as the respiratory infection improves. But the appendicitis may be genuine, brought on by this other infection swelling the child's glands.

So even if a child seems to have obvious signs of chest trouble, it is very important to tell the doctor if he or she also has a tummyache.

When to see the doctor
If the pain has continued for a whole day or night and has become increasingly severe, and if the patient is vomiting and unable to get up, then it is clearly time to seek medical help. It may be quicker to take the patient to the doctor's surgery, rather than wait for him to call. Home treatments, such as painkillers or soothing drinks should not be tried at this stage. An operation may be urgently needed, and the stomach must be empty of food and drink before an anaesthetic can be given.

Dangers of appendicitis
If the problem is neglected, the situation can become dangerous. The tip of the appendix can become gangrenous, causing perforation. If pus spreads into the abdominal cavity, the result can be a serious inflammation—called peritonitis —which can happen within hours. This can be localized in adults, but in children under 10, it can turn into general peritonitis. When the appendix is removed, a plastic drain has to be inserted to allow any infected matter to drain away. Intravenous fluids (a drip) and antibiotics will also be given to combat the infection and speed the child's recovery.

Appendectomy
Because the risks of neglecting appendi-

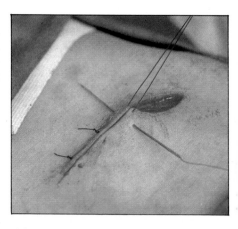

After an appendectomy the wound is carefully stitched so that only the smallest scar will remain.

citis are greater than the risks of an unnecessary operation, the surgeon will operate, even if in doubt. But, if the symptoms are inconclusive, the patient may be put to bed and kept under observation. If things do not improve, an operation will be performed.

The operation is quite simple and only takes about half an hour, under general anaesthetic. Modern drugs and antibiotics have greatly reduced the risk of complications. When the appendix has gone, the patient feels much better and is ready to leave hospital a few days later. The stitches at the site of the operation are removed after a week.

The healing process
Once the stitches have been taken out, the scar still has to heal but the patient can soon lead a reasonably normal life again, though active sports, like football or boxing are out of the question for several weeks.

After-effects
Occasional twinges of pain will be felt during the healing stage, but these will disappear within a month or so. However, the patient may develop severe wind a short time after the operation. This happens because the abdomen has been opened during surgery and air can enter the intestine when the appendix is removed.

Also, after any abdominal operation, the bowels cease working and so passing wind is a good sign because it shows that the digestive system is resuming its normal function—and this means that the patient can eat and drink again. So if patients feel any embarrassment, the best possible reassurance you can give is to point out that passing wind is a sign that their body is just getting back to normal and that they are well on the way to complete recovery.

Appetite

Q My young son is just getting over a bad cold and he doesn't want to eat anything. What can I do?

A Try to tempt him with foods he really likes. In fact, when any patient does not want to eat, there is not much that can be done apart from this. Fortunately, unless there is some reason why a person should not eat at all—it is possible to try any food. When someone really does not want to eat anything, one of the food substitute drinks you can buy should provide more than adequate nourishment until his normal appetite returns.

Q Is there some way I can know when I've eaten just enough—and stop over-eating?

A It is possible to become more aware of your body's signals, and, with practice, you can more accurately gauge how much food you really need. One way of finding out is to chew more slowly. This signals the appestat (the part of the brain which controls appetite) to stop you eating.

Q Why do I gain and lose weight during my menstrual cycle? Is this caused by food or by fluid retention?

A Some theories attribute this to an excess of body fluid caused by hormonal changes during the menstrual cycle. But a new theory states that the extra weight is gained because the hormones actually alter the appetite at this time, and the weight gain is a result of over-eating in response to this.

Q My husband says there is no reason for me to eat midday and evening—the evening meal is enough for him. Is he right?

A No. Our individual rhythms are controlled by hormones. They influence our sleeping and waking patterns as well as our eating habits and appetite. They help the brain to regulate the times at which we start and stop eating. Everyone's eating habits are, therefore, different as is the amount of food they require to give them energy.

If appetite and hunger were the same no one would be overweight or too thin—we would all eat the right amount to satisfy hunger and nourish ourselves. So what causes appetite and what is its purpose?

When you want to eat something because it looks good, smells nice and tastes delicious, your appetite is working. But when you want to eat something because your stomach is rumbling and you feel in need of food, then your hunger drive is working. This is the basic difference between appetite and hunger.

It is quite an important difference because it is not hunger that makes you overeat, but appetite. In the same way, although you might actually be hungry and need food, your appetite can stop you eating and so the body's needs are not satisfied. This happens in some diseases and in a condition such as anorexia nervosa, where the person becomes obsessed with dieting.

So, it seems that the body's way of letting us know our food requirements is via hunger. Also, it seems that appetite sometimes interferes, not letting the body get the right amount of nourishment. In this case, why do we have appetite, where does it come from, and are there times when it has a really useful role to play?

Developing an appetite
When a baby is born, one of the very first things he or she feels is the need for food. In most cases, this need is satisfied with milk, either from the mother's breast or from a bottle. At this stage in the baby's life, he or she shows no real preference for any type of food. The baby will cry when hungry and be calm and smiling when fed. It is only later that babies will learn what foods they really like.

With this learning, the growing child's appetites are gradually developed. It is because human beings are so complex that we have such different appetites and likes for different foods.

It is interesting to note that in countries that do not share our normal diet, things that we consider to be absolutely inedible are thought to be delicious delicacies. It is also quite revealing that in countries where there is starvation, people do not get the chance to exercise their appetites and are hungry enough to eat virtually anything to keep themselves alive.

How appetite works
Appetite is the regulator of our daily food intake, and thus the eventual regulator of how much we weigh. Because of this, many scientists are very interested in precisely what controls the appetite and they have found that it is quite a complicated process.

In most people, when the appetite is satisfied, eating stops. It is what causes this that is so interesting. It might seem obvious that when you are full you stop eating, but experiments have shown that it is not just a full stomach that tells the brain to stop. For instance, it has been found that there is a hormone produced by the intestines that signals the brain to stop eating.

Other signals come from the concentration of nutrients in the blood, the

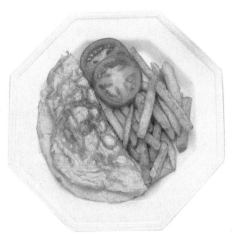

Colour and presentation have much to do with stimulating appetite. This food is nutritionally balanced and attractive.

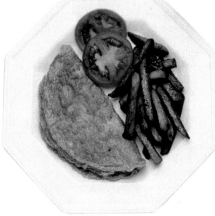

The same food coloured blue (the most unappetizing colour) and green is not likely to stimulate anyone's appetite.

Di Lewis

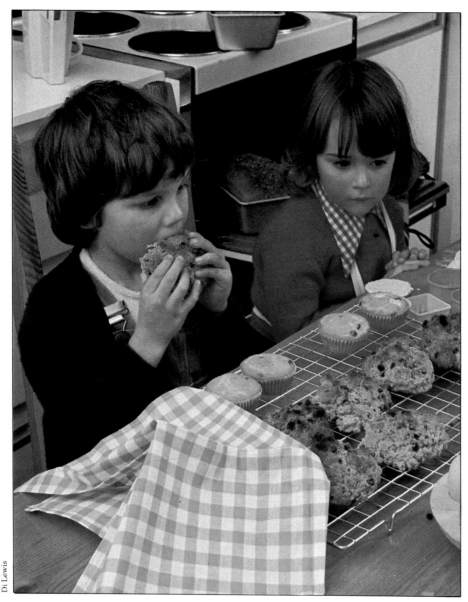

Di Lewis

The aroma of warm, freshly-baked bread and buns is sure to encourage children's appetites, particularly if they have helped to make them.

A normal weight person seems to care less about the food than the fact that he or she is taking in fuel to keep the body running. So, at mealtimes fat people will eat out of habit and eat more than they need, if the food tastes good, and normal weight people will eat only enough to satisfy their hunger, without really caring too much about what the food actually tastes like.

But, again, this does not take account of things like eating binges that all people who are overweight know about only too well. Also, people eat for a number of reasons that have nothing to do with food taste or the regularity of mealtimes. A lot of theories put forward say that people eat to compensate for some frustration or because they are bored and lonely. Everyone who has raided the fridge in the middle of the night will know that they are really doing it because they want to gain some sort of emotional satisfaction and comfort from the act of eating—and not to relieve any need for food.

amount of food that has passed through the mouth and the degree of fullness of the stomach. All these signals are picked up by an area of the brain called the hypothalamus.

Scientists have discovered that there are two separate areas in the hypothalamus that are in charge of eating. One of them controls eating and the other controls satiety, or satisfaction of appetite. The name given to these two areas together is the appestat.

So, all these signals go to the appestat and when there are enough from the areas that are concerned with eating, the appestat tells the brain that the body has had enough and eating stops. This all

sounds very simple, but, unfortunately, it does not always work quite like this. If it did, no one would be overweight or too thin, but this is obviously not the case. So what happens?

Fat and thin

One theory for this is that fat people, or those that eat more than they need, have an appestat that is set too high. In other words, the appestat does not tell the brain to stop eating soon enough.

The opposite is true for thin people: they stop eating too soon. But this theory does not take into account any of the other reasons for over or underweight.

It has been found that fat people are more likely to eat when they see food in front of them, while a person with normal weight will only eat when hungry. Also, fat people pay more attention to the taste of food.

Abnormal appetite

There are times in almost everyone's life when, for one reason or another, an abnormal appetite develops. This can be a time when less is eaten, more is eaten or even very unusual foods are eaten.

During illness, it is quite common for people to go off their food. At the moment there is no rational explanation as to why this happens, as often it is very much in the sick person's interests to eat properly. Doctors think that there might be subtle changes in the workings of the body that simply reduce both hunger and appetite.

Another common type of unusual appetite can happen during pregnancy. The stories of pregnant mothers eating all sorts of strange foods or combination of foods are legion. There is every likelihood that the hormone changes in early pregnancy actually change the sense of taste, making previously pleasant foods or drinks taste strange and unpalatable. The eating of very unusual things like coal and earth does not seem to be so common these days, and doctors think that this behaviour was caused by the mother needing to make up a mineral deficiency. In this case, the body appears to be cleverer than a lot of people think, as it can tell what unusual food to eat—to make up a deficiency—without the person knowing why.

Generally speaking, fads during pregnancy need not be a cause of anxiety. But a sick person who does not want to eat should be tempted with interesting dishes to take nourishment.

Arteries and artery disease

Q I have been told that smoking causes artery disease. Is this true?

A Yes. Hardening of the arteries (arteriosclerosis) is aggravated by smoking, although exactly how this happens is unclear. But there is no doubt that nicotine in the bloodstream does cause arteries to narrow. After a while, they become permanently rigid and less able to carry blood to all parts of the body, particularly the heart—resulting in heart attacks—and the extremities (hands and feet). If blood cannot reach the extremities, tissues degenerate, gangrene sets in, and a limb may have to be amputated.

However, if smoking is given up in time, damage can be avoided.

Q I jog regularly. Will this reduce the chance of my having a heart attack?

A There is a reasonable amount of evidence to suggest that regular exercise does have a protective effect against heart attacks, but this is by no means conclusive. A recent study comparing the chances of heart attacks among bus drivers with bus conductors showed a small difference in favour of the conductors, whose job is more active than the drivers'. So it seems reasonable to assume that exercise is a preventive measure and jogging a good idea.

Q Three of my male relatives, including my father, have died of heart attacks. Are men more prone to atheriosclerosis than women?

A This does appear to be so, for several reasons. Firstly, female hormones seem to protect women from atheroma (the build-up of fatty deposits in the arteries, which can cause blockages); after the menopause, with its fall in the level of hormone production, atheroma increases. Secondly, until recently, more men smoked than women, but now the pattern is altering and, as a result, the number of women suffering from atheroma before and after the menopause is rising. The conclusion is obvious: give up smoking.

The arteries carry blood containing nourishment and oxygen to all parts of the body. Artery disease is therefore very dangerous, so preventive measures are essential and early treatment vital.

The arteries and veins are the two sorts of large blood vessels in the body. The arteries are like pipes, carrying blood outwards from the heart to the tissues while the veins carry the blood on the return journey. The entire body depends on blood for its supply of oxygen and other vital substances without which life could not go on indefinitely.

The artery network
The heart is a pump which propels blood around the body through the arteries. The main pumping chamber on the left side of the heart, which is called the left ventricle, ejects blood into the main artery of the body – the aorta. The aorta is a tube about 2.5 cm across on the inside

The first of its branches arise from

The arterial system

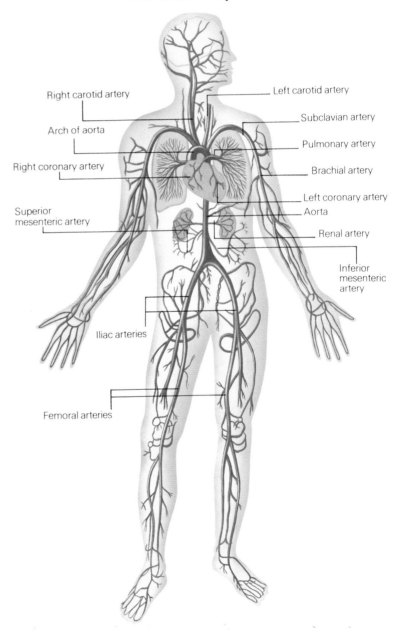

Right carotid artery

Arch of aorta

Right coronary artery

Superior mesenteric artery

Left carotid artery

Subclavian artery

Pulmonary artery

Brachial artery

Left coronary artery

Aorta

Renal artery

Inferior mesenteric artery

Iliac arteries

Femoral arteries

Venner Artists

Development of atherosclerosis

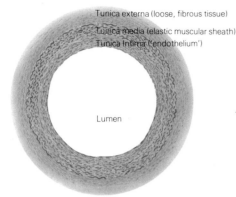
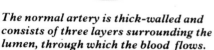

Tunica externa (loose, fibrous tissue)
Tunica media (elastic muscular sheath)
Tunica intima ('endothelium')

Lumen

Mike Courteney

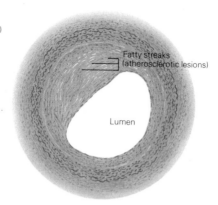

Fatty streaks
(atherosclerotic lesions)

Lumen

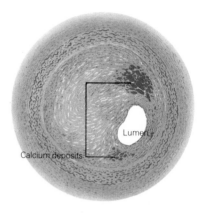

Lumen

Calcium deposits

The normal artery is thick-walled and consists of three layers surrounding the lumen, through which the blood flows.

In a moderate case of atherosclerosis, fatty deposits begin to be built up in the inner layer of the artery.

Here, atherosclerosis is almost total: fatty deposits have severely decreased the lumen and calcium is forming.

the aorta as soon as it leaves the heart. These are the coronary arteries which supply blood to the heart itself. The coronary arteries are particularly likely arteries to be affected by disease. A blocked coronary artery–or coronary thrombosis–causes a heart attack.

After giving rise to the coronary arteries, the aorta passes upward before doubling back on itself in an arch. Originating from this arch are the two main arteries to the head, the left and right carotid arteries, and one artery to each arm. The aorta descends down the chest and into the abdomen.

In the abdomen there are three main arteries to the intestines and the liver, and one to each kidney before the aorta divides into the left and right iliac arteries which supply blood to the pelvis and the legs.

After passing through the capillaries–a network of tiny blood vessels linking the smallest arteries and veins–from which oxygen and nourishment enter the tissues, the blood returns towards the heart in the veins. In general, the artery and vein supplying an area tend to run side by side. The veins empty into the right side of the heart, from where blood is pumped to the lungs and recharged with oxygen. From the lungs, oxygen-rich blood is drained by the pulmonary veins into the left side of the heart.

Here, it starts off round the body again by being pumped into the aorta by the left ventricle of the heart. The left ventricle generates a considerable pressure to force the blood through the arterial network. The tightness which the inflatable cuff used in taking blood-pressure around your arm reaches is the same as the maximum squeeze in the left ventricle with each heartbeat.

The structure of arteries

Since the arteries are subjected to this force with each heartbeat, they have to be thick-walled to cope with the pressure. The outer wall of an artery is a loose, fibrous tissue sheath. Inside this there is a thick elastic and muscular sheath which gives the artery its strength. There are also rings of muscle fibres encircling the artery in among the elastic tissue (the 'endothelium'). The inner layer of the artery is made of a smooth layer of cells which allows the blood to flow freely.

The thick elastic walls are most important to the way in which the system works. Much of the force of each heartbeat is taken up in the elastic walls of the big arteries. They continue to push the blood forward in the pause between each heartbeat.

Artery disease

Arterial disease in any part of the body is dangerous because if an artery is blocked or narrowed it is possible that the part it supplies will die from oxygen starvation. There are two basic ways in which a blockage can happen.

Hardening of the arteries is the commonest serious illness in the Western world. Age is the most important cause, but many other factors affect the rate at which arterial disease progresses.

The changes in the walls of arteries which lead to hardening are called arteriosclerosis ('sclerosis' means hardening). These changes are caused by the development of an excessive amount of fibrous tissue. This can happen as a result of straining of the artery walls caused by raised blood pressure.

The other type of disease is atheroma, which is the name given to fatty deposits which attach themselves to the arterial

walls increasingly with advancing age. These fatty deposits look like porridge and 'atheroma' is Greek for porridge.

Changes in the arterial network resulting from atheroma, as opposed to arteriosclerosis are usually referred to as atherosclerosis–a word your doctor is more likely to use than arteriosclerosis. Arterio–and atherosclerosis are words which can be used interchangeably.

Cholesterol

The atheromatous process first starts with a deposit of cholesterol–a normal constituent of the blood and one of the building blocks of normal cells–in the wall of the artery. However, it seems that cholesterol leaks into the inner surface (intima) of the artery and a 'fatty streak' forms within the arterial wall.

As the fatty streak grows in size and depth two other things happen. First, the surface of the streak may break down and expose the middle portions of the arterial wall to the blood. When this happens it triggers the mechanism for clotting the blood. A clot normally forms as a plug of fibrous tissue to stop bleeding from a wound. When the process occurs around a fatty streak, a mixture of fibrous and fatty tissue is formed in the arterial wall and this is called an atheromatous plaque. As the plaque grows it starts to encroach upon the central blood-filled space–that is, the lumen of the artery.

Finally, the development of the plaque involves changes occurring deep in the arterial wall. Fibrous tissue forms on the inner surface of the original fatty streak, but there is also a growth of fibrous tissue on the wall side of the plaque, growing from the outside of the artery towards its centre. The end result is a mixture of fibrous and fatty tissue blocking a proportion of the arterial lumen. The disease extends to a considerable depth in the wall of the vessel and encroaches on a large proportion of its circumference.

Once a large atheromatous plaque has formed it may have a number of consequences. It may steadily enlarge to block the artery. Because the artery is partially blocked, the flow of blood past the obstruction is reduced. This may activate the clotting system at the site of narrowing. The clot may well produce a complete obstruction known as a thrombosis. Atheromatous plaques which are partly blocking an artery may become displaced and swing across the lumen of the artery, like a lock gate, to block it completely. Parts of an atheromatous plaque may break off and travel towards a smaller artery which will then become blocked. This is a phenomenon known as embolism.

Atheroma can affect any artery down to a diameter of about 2 millimetres. However, the process is most likely to occur in areas of arterial wall which are subjected to movement and most stress. For this reason, atheroma is commonest at sites where arteries branch into smaller arteries. There is a greater stretching of the lining of the arteries at these points allowing more cholesterol to get into the wall.

The results of blockage

Since arteries are necessary to supply oxygen to every part of the body, there is no organ which is completely immune to the effects of arterial disease. If an organ or a limb has its blood supply cut off by atheroma then it must eventually die. An area of tissue which has lost its oxygen supply is called an area of infarction. When this process occurs in an arm or a leg it is more usual to use the term gangrene.

There are obviously some areas where the effects of atheroma cause especially severe problems. The most important are the heart, the brain, the legs and, finally, the aorta itself.

Heart attacks

Atheroma particularly affects the heart because the two coronary arteries, the arteries that supply blood to the heart, are under more mechanical stress than practically any other arteries in the body. The heart is continuously contracting and relaxing with each heartbeat and, in so doing, the coronary arteries, which lie on the outer surface of the heart, are alternately stretched and relaxed. This seems to give ideal conditions for atheromatous plaques to be formed. When a coronary artery becomes blocked as a result of atheroma, then a heart attack results. Such an event may also be

known as a coronary thrombosis, or a myocardial infarction (the 'myocardium' is the heart muscle and infarction is the formation of a dead area of the muscle when it is deprived of blood).

But heart attacks are not the only problem which atheroma causes in the heart. Where there is a fixed obstruction which is not totally blocking the artery, the supply of blood to the heart may only be sufficient to meet the needs of the body when at rest. Exercise increases the need for blood in the heart and it becomes starved of oxygen. This causes pain arising in the heart which is known as angina pectoris, or simply angina. The two problems of angina and myocardial infarction are often lumped together under the title of ischaemic heart disease, ischaemia being a word which implies a lack of oxygen without total deprivation or infarction.

Strokes

In the brain atherosclerosis may result in a stroke. These may vary from the trivial to the fatal and may occur as a result of an artery becoming blocked through atheroma or embolism or through an artery leaking blood into the brain as a result of a weakened wall.

When the legs are severely affected by atheroma they become painful and this pain is worse during exercise, just as with angina. If the disease is severe, then gangrene results and the affected leg may have to be amputated.

Finally, the aorta itself is a very important area of atheromatous disease. Two different things can happen. The

An arteriogram is an X-ray in which dye is injected into the bloodstream to detect blockages. This arteriogram of an upper leg is normal and shows no blockage.

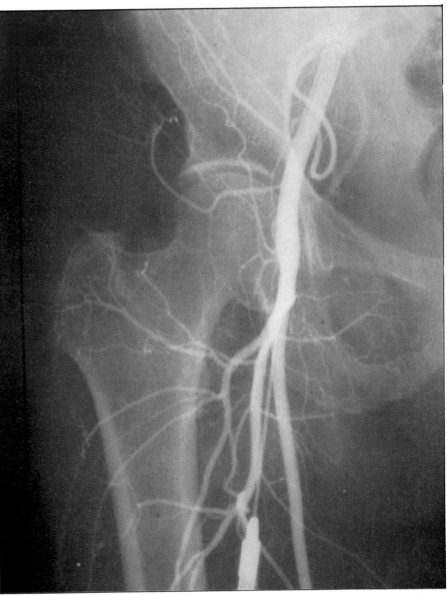

C James Webb

Q I know that smoking is bad for me. But will alcohol also increase the likelihood of my getting a bad heart?

A There is no evidence that moderate amounts of alcohol make atheroma worse; indeed, there are pointers in the opposite direction. Moderation, however, should still be observed. An excess is harmful in other ways.

Q I have arterial disease. Should I try and keep my legs warm?

A If you are suffering from peripheral vascular disease which reduces—and can prevent—blood flow to the extremities, you may be feeling the cold. Unfortunately, warming up your legs will only increase their demand for oxygen which is supplied by the blood. In hospital, legs badly afflicted by arterial disease are deliberately kept cool in the hope of preserving them. I should take further advice from your own doctor who knows the history of your condition.

Q My husband and I eat a lot of meat and dairy products. Do you think I should cut my husband's intake down, as I am worried about its cholestrol content?

A There are several very important points here. Firstly, if your husband smokes, there is no point in doing anything until he stops, as this will counteract the good effects of any other measures.

Secondly, you should be aware that there is more to a prudent diet than simply cutting down on cholesterol intake. Most of this comes from the body's own chemical processes anyway, and it is these that the prudent diet should aim to alter. It would seem sensible to move the diet towards more unrefined carbohydrate—that is, foods containing a lot of roughage like wholemeal bread and bran.

Then try and reduce all fats, in particular animal fats and dairy produce—called 'saturated fats', replacing them with those of vegetable origin. A diet such as this will reduce the intake of cholesterol while at the same time having a dramatic effect on the cholesterol already in the blood.

wall of the aorta may start to balloon out as a result of the weakening effect of the disease. This produces sack-like swelling called an aneurism instead of the regular tubular structure of the normal aorta. Aneurisms are usually found in the abdomen but may occur in the chest. An aneurism may continue to expand and eventually start to leak, with disastrous results. Surgical treatment is the only hope and it is necessary to strengthen the aorta with a woven fabric tube. The results of this sort of surgery when carried out as an emergency are often good, although there are failures.

Another form of aneurism which tends to occur in the chest rather than the abdomen, is called dissection of the aorta. This means that the layers of the aortic wall become split by escaping blood, the end result being much the same. Occasionally, patients survive dissection without surgery but, again, surgery is usually necessary.

Those affected

There is now a well-established list of risk factors which indicate people who are more likely to suffer from 'accelerated' or 'early' atheroma. For instance, some diseases put people at greater risk. The two most important are high blood pressure and diabetes.

People from a family in which atherosclerosis has occurred are at greater risk of developing problems themselves. And, finally, there is the cholesterol level in the blood. Although this is a definite risk factor, the value of cholesterol measurements in individuals has perhaps been overemphasized. However, it does seem sensible to reduce the amount of meat and dairy products in your diet.

Prevention

What can we do to prevent or postpone the development of atheromatous disease? Obviously both diabetes and high blood pressure must be treated. If there are no predisposing illnesses, then the most potent risk factor is family history, over which there is no control. However, there is one controllable factor left—smoking. The most effective thing to prevent atheroma is to stop smoking, for it can counteract the benefits of other measures. Apart from significantly reducing the chances of your developing heart disease, giving up cigarettes will generally improve your health.

This thermograph, or heat-sensitive picture, shows the effects of smoking on the circulation. Note the decreased blood flow to the fingertips.

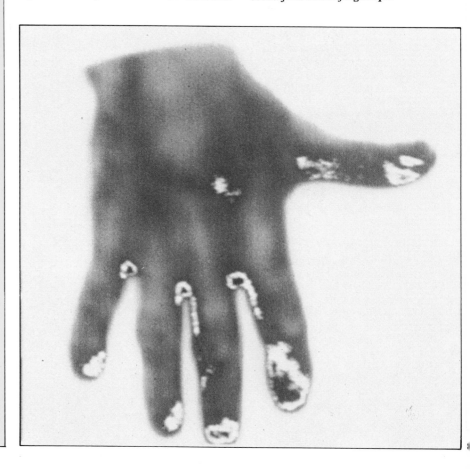

Arthritis

Q An old countryman once told me that he avoided arthritis by keeping a piece of cut potato in his pocket. Is there anything in this?

A You might as well believe that the moon is made of green cheese! Although many herbs have proven medicinal properties, the potato is not one of them. Your friend was just lucky enough not to have developed arthritis.

Q Is it safe to take a lot of aspirin to ease pain caused by arthritis?

A Yes and no. Because aspirin reduces inflammation and temperature and eases pain, it is often used as a first-line treatment for arthritis. Unfortunately, there are two side-effects that can happen when aspirin is taken for a long time. Bleeding can start from tiny gastric ulcers or an existing ulcer can flare up. If you start vomiting blood, or something that looks like coffee grounds, or pass black, tar-like bowel motions—stop taking the aspirin and seek medical help. The risk of stomach upsets is greatly reduced if you always use soluble aspirin. Another side effect is ringing in the ears—if this happens, reduce the amount of aspirin.

Q Are some occupations more likely to cause arthritis than others?

A Regrettably, yes. Doctors are familiar with various 'wear and tear' effects, such as 'baker's cyst'—which is fluid at the back of the knee produced by excessive bending (when getting bread in and out of the oven), 'porter's neck'—which is osteoarthritis of the neck joints, caused by tilting the neck (when carrying objects over the shoulder), and even 'ballet dancer's toe'—which looks like a bunion.

Q Can I do any good to an inflamed joint if I rub liniment on it?

A Very little, but you may find it soothing. Vegetable oil or soap liniment are cheapest and as good as anything. For a bruised joint, massage with emollients may help.

Many people are affected by some form of arthritis, which can range from temporary discomfort to a more serious disability, but medical help and physiotherapy can do much to relieve the condition.

Arthritis is an inflammation of the joints and its causes are as varied and mysterious as the condition itself. It affects people of all ages and is a common complaint in temperate climates; it can be mild or severe, affecting one joint or several; and the different types include rheumatoid arthritis, osteoarthritis, rigid spine disease (*ankylosing spondylitis*) and arthritis that has been brought on by an injury or other infection. Although its study is a well-established speciality, called rheumatology, medical research cannot yet tell us all the answers.

Rheumatoid arthritis in adults

Although it is common, the cause of rheumatoid arthritis is unknown. It is thought that it may be due to an 'auto-immune' phenomenon—that is, some event, perhaps a severe illness or a shock which triggers a chain of chemical reactions within the body. eventually producing chemicals which react against the body's own tissues–in this case, against the lining tissue of the joints–the

This X-ray shows a badly diseased arthritic hip. Suitable treatment would be hip joint replacement.

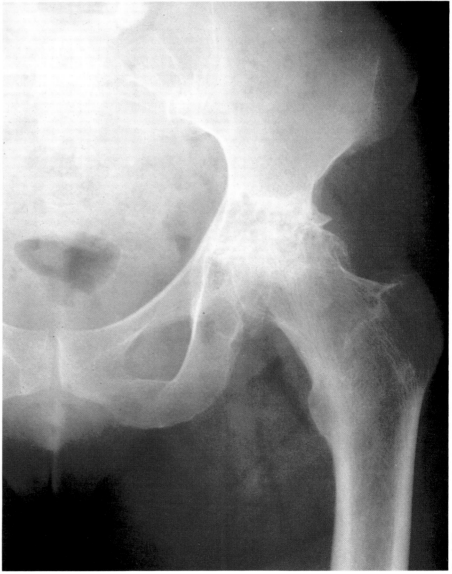

Derek Ellis

synovium. Inflammation and arthritis will follow.

Rheumatoid arthritis usually affects adults between the ages of 20 and 55, and women are three times more liable to it than men. Inflammation of the knuckles of both hands is the usual symptom, and the joints of the toes are affected in a similar way. At the same time, the sufferer may lose weight, feel unwell and become lethargic. The symptoms may be either acute, starting with a fever or rash, or happen gradually over several weeks.

The joints most often affected are the knees, hips, shoulders, wrists, elbows, ankles and the bones of the neck. The stiffness is usually at its worst in the mornings, and in acute cases the sufferer may be confined to bed or have great difficulty with movement.

In about one quarter of cases, attacks will last about six months, but only happen every few years. Some cases are persistent, varying in severity, but tending to 'burn out' after many years.

In children

Rheumatoid arthritis can occur in children—a condition called Still's disease—but it is fortunately rare. Two main age groups are affected—between one and three and 10 and 15. The inflammation starts gradually, and in about one third of cases occurs in one joint

only, commonly the knee. It can also affect the hands, wrists, feet and ankles.

This disease is slowly progressive, but burns itself out in late adolescence. The chances of a cure depend on the severity of the case, how early it is diagnosed and how quickly treatment is begun. It should be started early to prevent permanent stiffening and joint deformity .

Osteoarthritis

Osteoarthritis occurs as part of the ageing process. It happens mainly to weight-bearing joints: hips, knees and spine. In women the hands are also often affected, particularly the top joints of the fingers and the base of the thumb.

This condition is caused by a degeneration of the cartilage, a tough, elastic tissue which protects the surface of the joint. This is normally glistening and smooth, but osteoarthritis causes it to roughen and the cartilage becomes 'dry'. This change has two effects: it compresses the underlying bone surface that the **cartilage should protect** and inflames the synovium (the lining) lying over it.

The first symptoms are pain and loss of use; stiffness and swelling follow, and the joint eventually changes shape. There may be only one joint involved, such as the right hip in a right-handed person (because right-handedness means that the right side of the body is more active

and bears more weight then the left), or, in many cases, the knees, spine, shoulders, hands and neck are affected. This condition is also slowly progressive, but disability rarely happens unless the arthritis in a weight-bearing joint is severe. Unfortunately, any injury will cause the condition to flare up.

Rigid spine disease

Ankylosing spondylitis is a form of arthritis which affects the pelvic joints and spine. This, too, is thought to be an auto-immune illness, like rheumatoid arthritis, but there is a definite tendency for it to run in families. It is more common in men, usually starting between the ages of 15 and 30.

The inflammation causes calcium to be deposited in the ligaments (fibrous bands which connect joints). This results in stiffness which can lead to the spinal bones (the vertebrae) being fused together if the inflammation is not alleviated by both medical treatment and exercise—hence its colloquial name 'poker back'. The illness progresses slowly for a few years, often spreading to the whole spine and involving the hip joints, before gradually petering out.

Other causes of arthritis

An injury can trigger arthritis—this is called 'traumatic' arthritis. The injury

Comparison of a normal and an osteoarthritic knee joint

In osteoarthritis some cartilage, which lines the bones of the knee joint, forms into lumps (osteophytes) and some wears away. As it wears, bones lose their protection which causes pain.

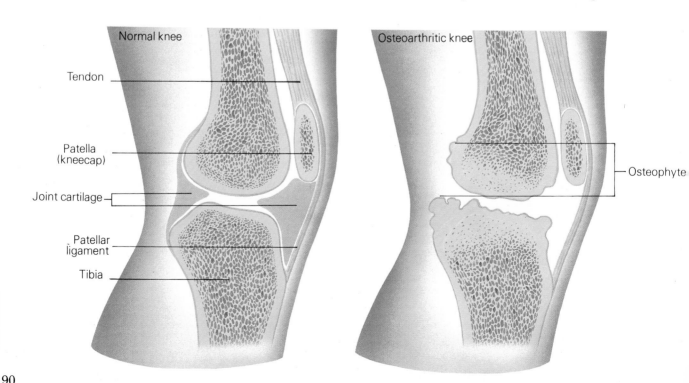

Normal knee

Tendon
Patella (kneecap)
Joint cartilage
Patellar ligament
Tibia

Osteoarthritic knee

Osteophyte

Mike Courteney

Types of arthritis and their treatment

Type	Cause	Symptoms	Treatment
Rheumatoid arthritis	'Auto immune', i.e. chain of reactions in body	Lethargy, high temperature, rash (occasionally)	Anti-inflammatory drugs, painkilling drugs, gold injections or steroid drugs. Immediate hospital treatment for children. Reducing swelling by drawing off (aspirating) fluid, physiotherapy, exercise, splinting, joint replacement
	Affects adults between 20 & 55 also children (Still's disease)	Pain, swelling, redness, stiffness and loss of function in joints of fingers or toes.	
Osteoarthritis	Wear and tear due to ageing; degeneration of cartilage over joint	Pain, followed by stiffness, swelling, change of shape	Basic principles as above
Ankylosing spondylitis	'Auto immune'—possibly hereditary, more common in males between 15 & 30, calcium deposited in joint ligaments	Stiff lower back in mornings, pain on bending spine	Anti-inflammatory drugs, exercise
Traumatic	Injury ,e.g. falling heavily	Joint becomes inflamed, painful and swollen a few hours after injury	Rest, bandaging, painkilling drugs, then physiotherapy. X-ray in case of fracture, possible aspiration of fluid

can either be direct, for example from a blow to a joint, or indirect, as when you hurt your knee by falling heavily on it. Traumatic arthritis usually happens to men, although no-one is immune.

The knee, ankle or wrist are the joints most-commonly affected. A few hours after the injury, the joint becomes inflamed, painful and swollen. An X-ray is needed, in case a fracture has occurred, but rest, bandaging and painkillers may be all that is necessary.

Physiotherapy can also help restore mobility and muscle power to the affected limb. Occasionally the injury causes bleeding into the joint which becomes very tense and painful; this may have to be drawn out with a needle (aspirated) under a local anaesthetic.

Germs can also cause conditions like septic arthritis, which is brought on by a germ in the joint fluid. This happens either because of an injury or because it is transmitted from the blood. Half of such cases involve the knee, but it can occur in any large joint. Both children and the elderly can be affected, but it is fortunately rare.

Another rare form of arthritis can result from an attack of German measles (rubella). This can happen to adults, who may experience swelling of their finger joints, knees and ankles which subsides after a few weeks.

Arthritis of the lower spine and hip, resulting from tuberculosis, is now also rare except in people from the developing countries. Other infections such as rheumatic fever, gonorrhoea and the skin disease psoriasis, can also give rise to arthritis.

Diagnosis and treatment
If you suspect that you have some form of arthritis, the worst thing you can do is to 'just put up with it'. Do not try to make the diagnosis yourself, but go and see your doctor. Any delay might mean the risk of permanent deformity, especially in the case of a child with Still's disease, a condition which needs hospital care.

Your doctor will ask for a history of your illness and give you an examination. He may prescribe drugs such as aspirin, indomethacin and ibuprofen, which combat inflammation and ease pain, and painkillers like paracetamol or distalgesic tablets, which are stronger. Gold injections may be given in the affected joints, but these can have unpleasant side-effects and are used only when absolutely necessary.

You may have to rest the affected joints or wear an individually-made splint to keep them in the best position and so prevent deformities from occurring. Swelling in joints can be treated by

Coping with arthritis at home

● Build ramp to replace outdoor steps.

● Make door openings wide enough to take wheelchair, if necessary.

● Fix handrail on both sides of stairs

● Replace worn carpets; keep floor space clear for walking aids.

● Raise electric sockets about 1m (3 ft) above ground.

● Replace light switches with pull cords.

● Fix wire basket inside door below letter box to save bending.

● Raise heights of chairs with blocks fixed to ends of chair legs; raise height of seat with firm cushions.

● To increase leverage on refrigerator handle, slip loop of leather, or strong string over handle.

● Pad handles of utensils (e.g. potato peeler) with foam rubber; also brush and broom handles.

● Use basket on wheels to carry things from one room to another.

● Fix handrails to bath and around toilet; raised toilet seat.

● Iron and ironing board fixed to wall to avoid carrying.

● Electric 'ripple' bed-current ripples through plastic mattress to give cushioning effect.

● Long-handled garden tools.

● Adjustable seat in bath.

● Lightweight carpet sweeper.

● Extend toilet seat for wheelchair users.

● Washing machine and kitchen surfaces at convenient heights.

Q My doctor says I have a 'frozen shoulder'. Is that a form of arthritis?

A No. It is simply a condition that mimics it. Others in this category include 'tennis elbow' and nerve-pain in the wrist, which is called carpal tunnel syndrome. What these conditions have in common is inflammation of the tissues around a joint—but in each case, other evidence confirming arthritis is absent.

Q My daughter is severely affected by arthritis but she is planning to get married in the very near future. What are her chances of enjoying any sex life or starting a family?

A When either partner has arthritis, they will want answers to many questions before they start a family. An important point is whether their children will be especially prone to this condition. Only one type of arthritis, caused by haemophilia is clearly inherited. With many other forms the chances of an affected parent handing on the disease are rare. In an acute phase of the disease, it would be painful to attempt sex, but otherwise it is quite safe to have intercourse.

Q My grandmother always wears a bandage on her arthritic knee. Is this really helpful?

A Bandaging or supporting an acutely inflamed joint can stop any jarring movement and therefore ease pain. When a joint is swollen, the tissues feel stretched—a support in these circumstances gives a sensation of stability. Wearing a bandage also serves to warn other people that a knock would *not* be appreciated!

Q I've been told heat is good for arthritis and am wondering if I could use an infra-red lamp to ease the pain?

A Heat is soothing and infra-red is a penetrating heat. Place it about 60cm (24in) away from the affected joint and use it for about 20 minutes—up to three times daily. There is no long-term benefit, but it can be useful if done just before you begin an exercise routine.

drawing off excess fluid under a local anaesthetic, or injecting an anti-inflammatory drug into the joint.

You may be feeling generally unwell and be advised to cut down some of your everyday activities and rest as much as possible. Steroid drugs (such as cortisone) may be prescribed to suppress the inflammation in the joints, but because they have side-effects they will only be used when all other forms of treatment have been unsuccessful. Doses must always be kept at the lowest possible level at which they will control symptoms, and progress must be carefully monitored by a doctor. fully monitored by a doctor.

If your symptoms persist, your doctor may recommend a visit to the rheumatic clinic of your local hospital for further investigation. An acute attack of arthritis with fever, swollen joints and a general feeling of being unwell may need immediate hospital treatment, including splinting and rest on a special 'ripple' bed—an electric current 'ripples' through a plastic mattress, giving a cushioning effect.

Blood tests are made to establish the

type of arthritis involved, to see if you are anaemic, to check the amount of inflammation in the body at regular intervals and to assess the progress of the disease. Other tests will show whether the condition is caused by septic arthritis, gonococcal (VD) arthritis, or by bleeding into the joint.

Another technique, called arthroscopy, involves a telescope-type instrument which is used to look inside the knee joint under local anaesthetic. Both the cartilage and lining tissue can be examined by this means, and small pieces of tissue can be removed for further microscopic examination to help establish the cause of the condition.

Exercise and physiotherapy

Physiotherapy plays an important part in the treatment of all forms of arthritis. For affected joints that are in a 'quiescent' phase—that is, free of inflammation, exercise is essential to prevent stiffness and loss of mobility and restore muscles around the joint that may have wasted. There is no evidence that exercising an arthritic joint in the quiescent phase

In this adapted kitchen the emphasis is on areas which ensure the maximum of *ease and efficiency for arthritics when using their hands or bending.*

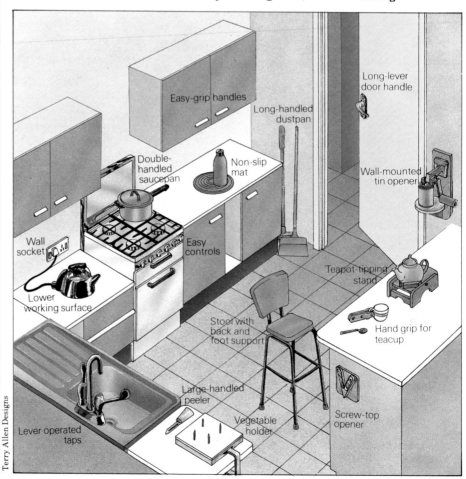

Easy-grip handles
Long-lever door handle
Long-handled dustpan
Non-slip mat
Double-handled saucepan
Wall-mounted tin opener
Wall socket
Easy controls
Teapot-tipping stand
Lower working surface
Stool with back and foot support
Hand grip for teacup
Large-handled peeler
Screw-top opener
Lever operated taps
Vegetable holder

Terry Allen Designs

Especially important in this bathroom are adaptations that allow the arthritis sufferer to sit comfortably and without too much bending. Note also the toilet flush which can be pressed and the lever taps in the bathtub.

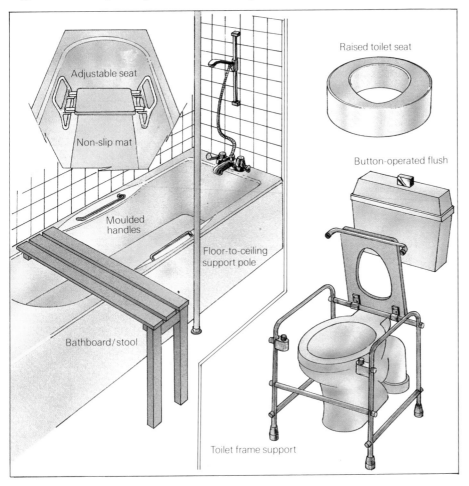

there is no cure yet for every disability caused by arthritis, better general care and physical aids can make life more tolerable in many ways.

Aids such as splints, surgical collars, walking sticks and frames, elbow crutches, wheelchairs and some of the more complicated electrical hoisting aids can all be matched to the individual needs by physiotherapists.

Advice can also be obtained from rehabilitation centres about specialized aids to mobility, such as electric wheelchairs.

Replacing one kind of lifestyle with another is always possible, although not always easy. Adjusting your employment must obviously take priority. You may need to change shifts, use specially adapted equipment or generally take on lighter duties. You doctor can help by writing to your employer about your specific problems.

Structural changes in the home may be necessary and there are many helpful adaptations that can be made. Living on one level in a bungalow or apartment is obviously more practical than living in a conventional two-storey house—but where this is not possible the problems caused by steps can be overcome by using special equipment. Nor need hobbies and pastimes as varied as card playing, gardening or needle craft be forgotten. Occupational therapists can advise about the many ingenious devices and techniques that have been developed to enable arthritics to continue enjoying these pleasures.

causes it to flare up.

The physiotherapist at your local hospital will teach you exercises which can be continued at home. Heat can be used to ease painful joints. These treatments can include short-wave diathermy, when a heater pad is placed near the affected joint, or hydrotherapy (exercising in a small, very warm swimming pool). The effect of the heat is to relax tense muscles and, because the water supports the weight of the body, movement is increased.

If your doctor or physiotherapist advises it, an infra-lamp can be used at home. Paraffin wax baths for hands and feet is another treatment that can be used very easily at home once the technique is learned. On the other hand, some therapists favour ice packs as a form of pain-relieving therapy.

The benefits of surgery
Great advances have been made in the replacement of badly-damaged joints with artificial ones. In the first place, the decision that an arthritic joint needs

surgery will be made by a specialist in the field, an orthopaedic surgeon who has been consulted by either the patient's doctor or a rheumatologist. The results of such an operation can be a dramatic relief of pain, correction of deformity and increased movement. The benefits to the patient may include restoring enjoyment of sexual intercourse which may have previously been very difficult.

Surgery can also relieve pressure around a joint, free gummed-up ligaments or remove the inflamed lining tissue of a joint (synovectomy) if it is excessively inflamed. An excruciatingly painful and useless joint such as may occur with osteoarthritis of the cervical spine (neck) or an arthritic knee is sometimes surgically fused (arthrodesis) to give relief, though this does involve loss of movement.

Help available
An active person, who has become seriously disabled, must first come to terms with the feelings of dependence and helplessness that this brings. Although

A physiotherapist helps the victim of arthritis with exercises and techniques such as heat treatment or hydrotherapy.

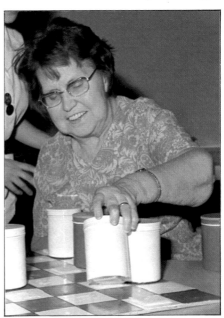

John Watney

Artificial insemination

Artificial insemination may seem a radical solution to an infertility problem, but it is in fact a simple medical technique which has enabled many couples to become parents who would otherwise be childless.

Q I have been married for several years and have not become pregnant. After tests on us both, our doctor has suggested artificial insemination, but I am worried that it will affect our marriage.

A Generally, AIH puts very little strain on a marriage—although some men can feel a sense of failure. However, both you and your husband should realize that he really will be the father of the child and that you can now have the baby you both long for. But if there are already stresses in a marriage, AID should not be undertaken. A husband's disappointment that he cannot be the father of the child, or a wife's resentment at not being able to have a natural child, can be enough to destroy a marriage. So it is very important that any such conflicts are resolved first.

Q If I have a child by artificial insemination will it be legitimate?

A A child conceived through AIH is legitimate. The legal position of a child conceived through AID varies from country to country; sometimes a child conceived in this way is not considered legitimate until the parents adopt it.

Q We have decided to try to have a child by AIH but are worried that it won't work. What is the success rate for artificial insemination?

A It varies, depending on the fertility of the woman, but, generally speaking, there is a success rate of between 50 and 70 per cent. However, it may be necessary to carry out the treatment for a period of six months to a year before it results in the desired pregnancy.

Q Is it possible that I will be able to choose the sex of my child if I conceive it by artificial insemination?

A No. It is no more possible for you to choose the sex of a child you conceive by artificial insemination than it is if you conceive a child during intercourse.

The term artificial insemination refers to the process in which sperm is inserted into the female reproductive tract by artificial means rather than through sexual intercourse. The sperm is usually placed next to the woman's cervix (the opening to the womb) using a syringe to which a long tube is attached.

Although increasingly used in cases of infertility, artificial insemination is one of several treatments available when couples fail to conceive. After carrying out tests, a couple's doctor will advise them on whether hormone treatment, surgery or artificial insemination will be the best treatment for them and will explain what is involved.

There are two forms of artificial insemination. If a woman has her husband's sperm inserted into her vagina, the process is called artificial insemination-husband (AIH). However, if the sperm of a different male is inserted, it is called artificial insemination-donor (AID).

Artificial insemination-husband

This method is used when there is some fault with the way the sperm is deposited in the vagina during normal intercourse. It may also be used to overcome some female reproductive problems.

For example, AIH might be used when there is some abnormality in the structure of the penis—a surprising number of men have the opening, which is usually found at the tip of the penis, situated elsewhere along the penile shaft. Most common of these conditions is where the opening is on the underside, back from the tip. So instead of the sperm being deposited next to the cervix, where they can easily swim up to meet the female eggs in the fallopian tubes, they are deposited nearer the entrance of the vagina and conception does not take place. However, by using artificial insemination, the sperm can be placed directly next to the cervix and so increase the chances of conception.

Another case might be when a man is unable to achieve an erection or when he is unable to ejaculate within the vagina. These men may be able to maintain strong erections and have ejaculations when masturbating, or through manual manipulation by the partner or in oral sex, but they lose these abilities as soon as penetration is attempted.

For men who have low sperm counts, a technique called *split ejaculate insemination* is used, which also involves AIH. When the sperm count is low, the number of sperm in the semen that has been ejaculated may be too low for fertilization to occur. However, the first part of the ejaculate always contains more sperm than the rest and if the first parts of several separate ejaculations are put together, then the number of sperm

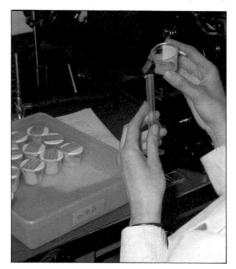

A labelled sample of recently ejaculated sperm is being tested for volume before being classified.

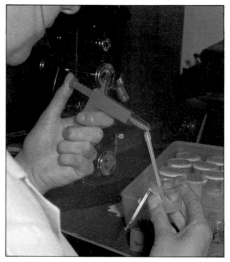

The sample is being diluted with a saline (salt water) solution as a preparation for the taking of a sperm count.

increases. Using AIH, this collection of several ejaculates is introduced into the woman at the time when she is most likely to conceive.

AIH can also be used when the barrier to conception is found in the female partner. For sperm to be able to enter the womb and swim up to fertilize the egg *(ovum)*, they must swim through the right quantity of watery mucus secreted by the cervix: some women produce too little mucus; others produce mucus so thick that the sperm cannot penetrate. AIH may solve this by attempting to put the sperm beyond the barrier.

Most parents tend not to tell the offspring that he or she was conceived through the use of AIH. In fact there is little to be gained by doing so. Besides, most parents usually forget the experience after several years.

Artificial insemination-donor

AID is used when the woman has no reproductive problems but either the man is sterile or the female is allergic to her partner's sperm. In this case, sperm is obtained from an unidentified male and introduced into the female in the same way that it is for AIH.

AID presents a good alternative, allowing a woman to have the experience of carrying and bearing a child which at least inherits *her* characteristics. And, since AID will be used only as a last resort to solve the problem of childlessness, most men feel quite happy about it.

The greatest care is taken in matching the donor's physical characteristics, such as height, build and complexion, with those of the husband, so that the child has the greatest chance of looking like both parents. The donors are also matched for

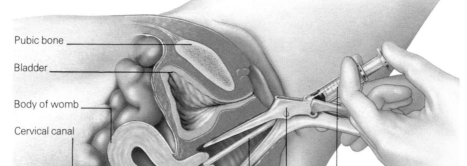

Artificial insemination by syringe

Pubic bone

Bladder

Body of womb

Cervical canal

Bowel

Syringe

Speculum

Plastic tube

Semen

Frank Kennard

intellectual ability.

The donors' medical and family histories are also examined carefully to avoid passing on conditions like diabetes or other inherited ailments. Furthermore, the characteristics of the female partner are also considered. If she does not have the Rh factor in her blood, for example, then a Rh negative donor is used to avoid future complications in pregnancy.

The matching procedures used are so effective that relatives, friends and the child itself do not generally suspect that AID has been used. But, in any case, genetic makeup of the offspring is far less important in the relationship between parents and child than genuine love.

Some doctors mix in some of the

In artificial insemination a warmed speculum (gynecological instrument) opens the vagina while a plastic tube carries the sperm sample from the syringe into the cervical canal.

husband's sperm with that of the donor (except where the woman reacts against her partner's sperm). This provides a small chance that the one sperm to penetrate could, after all, have come from the husband.

Research has shown that the children conceived by artificial insemination show no difference in rates of abnormality than children conceived in any other way.

The treatment

Treatment is carried out at infertility

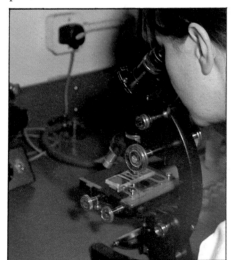

When it has been prepared, the sperm count itself is done under a very high powered microscope.

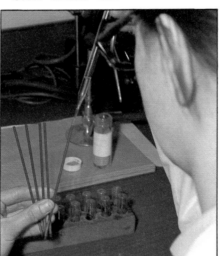

After all the tests have been carried out, the sample is dropped into pipettes (fine glass tubes) just before it is frozen.

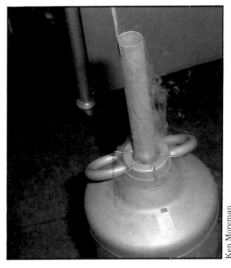

Prepared sperm is frozen in low-temperature liquid (liquid nitrogen) inside this sperm bank.

Ken Moreman

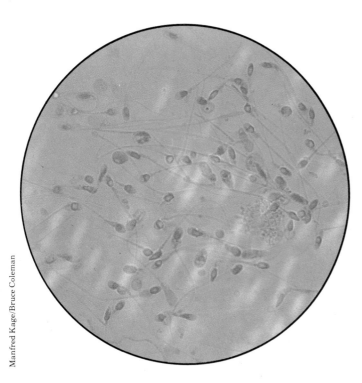

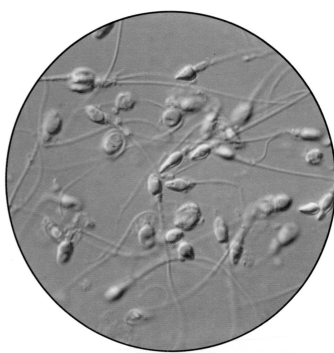

Manfred Kage/Bruce Coleman

clinics attached to gynaecological departments in some of the larger hospitals.

The first session in all cases of infertility consists of an interview with both partners. A medical examination is given to the woman, and a full medical and surgical history is obtained from both the man and the woman. Their attitudes towards one another, towards their infertility and towards children are also carefully discussed.

After this initial joint interview, the couple are usually examined separately: the woman has a gynaecological examination and a swab from her cervix is taken, and the man undergoes a full examination including his genitals.

Over successive sessions at the clinic, the doctors will establish the cause of the infertility. The man will always have to undergo a sperm count to help them do this, which involves giving a fresh specimen of semen. If the man feels he could not 'masturbate to order' at the clinic, he can produce his specimen at home, provided the sample is received at the hospital laboratory within two hours of ejaculation.

Sometimes the man may not be able to ejaculate through masturbating at all. In this case he is encouraged to have intercourse with his partner, but instead of ejaculating into her vagina, he does so into a dry, wide-mouthed jar kept ready by the bed.

The woman will be asked to monitor her basal body temperature—her temperature at rest before she begins any activity—since this provides clues as to

Normal sperm under the microscope (above left) and (above right) magnified 1000 times. A great number of sperms in any ejaculate, however, are abnormal and in many cases will not be able to swim properly: (right, top) this sperm has a head which is too large and a tail that is too short; (centre) this sperm's head is too large and its tail is double; (bottom) this sperm is grossly abnormal.

when ovulation is likely to be occurring. This is the time of the month when an egg is released from her ovary and she is at her most fertile. Once the cause of infertility is discovered and artificial insemination considered, the insemination can be arranged to take place at the times of ovulation to increase the chance of conception.

Artificial insemination is generally carried out on three consecutive days around the time of ovulation and may continue for a period of six months to a year. The sperm sample from either the husband or the donor is passed along a tube and inserted into the cervical canal. Where there is a cervical abnormality or a problem with the cervical mucus then the sample may be placed past the cervix within the uterus.

The sperm does not have to be fresh—provided it is frozen quickly following ejaculation, very little deterioration occurs. Indeed many men who undergo vasectomy (male sterilization) have samples of their sperm stored in sperm banks, and these samples have produced healthy children by artificial insemination.

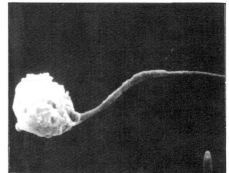

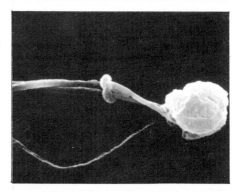

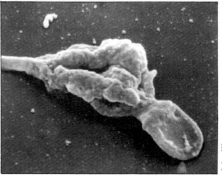

John Watney

Artificial limbs

Q I recently lost my leg in a car accident and am to be fitted with an artificial limb. I am frightened that it will feel peculiar and painful. Are my fears justified?

A An artificial leg is designed so that its socket fits the 'stump' of the natural limb comfortably. However, weight loss or gain will affect the fit of socket and stump and make the leg less comfortable to wear. If this happens, return to the hospital where the limb was fitted.

The wearing of an artificial limb can sometimes cause sensations of 'phantom pain' and of having a 'phantom limb'. Someone experiencing the latter knows exactly where the natural limb should be even though it is no longer there. To guard against 'phantom limb' it is important for sections of the artificial limb to be placed where the wearer feels they should be.

A small number of people who undergo amputation feel 'phantom pain'—that is, pain in the limb that is no longer there. The cause of the sensation is still being researched.

Q Does the wearing of an artificial limb cause any unpleasant odour?

A The socket of the artificial limb fits very closely to the stump of the natural one, and at the place where they meet the body may perspire. There will be no unpleasant smell of sweat if the wearer of the artificial limb is careful about personal hygiene, about keeping the limb itself thoroughly clean and about wearing a 'stump sock', which can be washed daily.

Q My son was born with one arm and needs an artificial limb. Will it be heavier than a natural limb and tire him out?

A The weight of an artificial limb is only about one-fifth of that of a natural limb, but because the latter is totally attached to the body, its weight is not obvious. A light but badly fitting artificial limb may feel heavier than one that is actually heavier but well fitting because the wearer will be conscious of it. So you need not be anxious about the weight of your son's artificial arm—if it is properly fitted it will not tire him.

Modern artificial limbs are highly efficient, comfortable and inoffensive to look at—and they are specially adapted to meet the individual needs of wearers.

An artificial limb is the product of highly skilled design and engineering, based on detailed and constantly improving research into the structure of the human frame and the movements of which it is capable, from walking and running to the slightest bending of a finger joint.

This limb must not simply fill the gap left by a missing natural limb or part of a limb, but must work comfortably and efficiently, so that it is as complete a replacement as possible, in both appearance and function.

Care in design
Amputation or the malformation of a natural limb at birth may cause the need for an artificial limb. Whatever the reason for it, it will be made according to precise and detailed information about the person who will use it: about age, height, weight and the general structure of the body, balance, skin colour and the way in which the person customarily makes movements and gestures.

The design of the limb will also take into consideration the way of life of the person concerned, particularly in terms of work and the things he or she enjoys doing in leisure time.

Comfort and efficiency
However well an artificial limb may be designed, its success as a useful addition to the body will obviously depend upon the attitude of the person who uses it. This in turn depends mainly upon two things: comfort and acceptance.

The design of modern, natural-looking artificial limbs takes into account all aspects of a person's life.

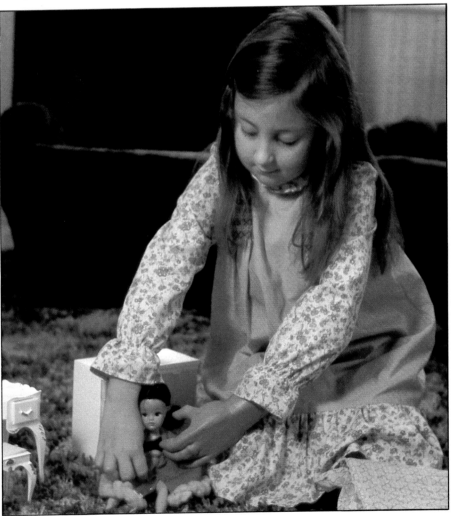

'Mother' Magazine

It is essential for an artificial limb to be comfortable. In its design and construction, great care is taken to ensure that the remaining part of the natural limb (the 'stump') and the 'socket' of the artificial one fit together smoothly. If there is no irritation or awkwardness in movement, the new limb will be accepted and become thoroughly useful much more quickly.

Good design and construction can do a great deal to make an artificial limb comfortable to wear and to use. How well it functions in use depends, first and foremost, upon a very detailed study of human movement, gesture and general physical behaviour.

Complexity of movement

It is easier to replace certain parts of the body with artificial limbs than others. The hand, for example, can make many small, delicate gestures; an artificial hand cannot, by itself, carry out more than a few of them, but is so constructed that a whole range of skilfully designed devices can be fitted to it so that the wearer can carry out precise and complex movements, such as those involved in driving a car.

The movements of the hip and knee are, by comparison with those of the hand, much more restricted, and an artificial limb can therefore replace them so accurately that the person wearing it will move in a natural way.

Training

No matter how well an artificial limb is designed, it can only function successfully if the person using it accepts it without fear or embarrassment and finds satisfaction in making it work to the full extent of its design. Both acceptance and adeptness depend, to some extent, on training. Anyone who needs to wear an

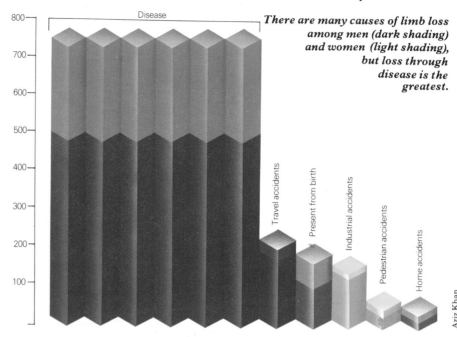

Causes of limb loss in the UK within one year

Disease

There are many causes of limb loss among men (dark shading) and women (light shading), but loss through disease is the greatest.

Travel accidents

Present from birth

Industrial accidents

Pedestrian accidents

Home accidents

Aziz Khan

artificial limb—and there are many thousands of people who do—can have expert help from specially trained staff in a number of major hospitals.

An artificial limb is an addition to the body, something imposed upon it, often after the shock of amputation, and the person who wears it must have time and

encouragement to grow accustomed to it in his thoughts and emotions as well as to use it to its best advantage and without self-consciousness.

This car has been specially adapted for a thalidomide victim. Note the steering wheel extended to reach her arms.

This detail of the car shows the modified control panel fitted into the right-hand door for ease of movement.

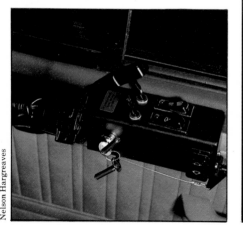

Nelson Hargreaves

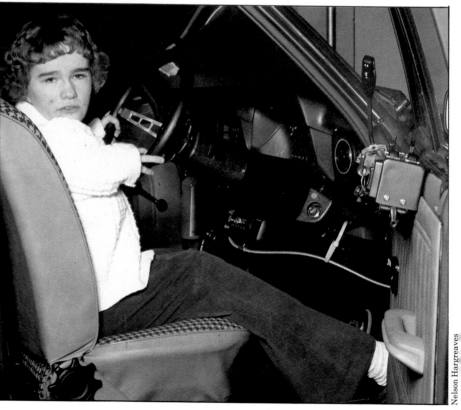

Nelson Hargreaves

Artificial respiration

Q Could I be asphyxiated if I fell asleep in front of my gas fire and the flame went out?

A Unfortunately this is possible, although the likelihood depends on the size of your room. As the air in the room becomes filled with gas, the amount of oxygen reaching your lungs will decrease. In the end you would become unconscious and die. To help prevent an accident like this, never sleep in front of the fire if it is on a low flame and make sure your room is draught-proof. Alternatively, use an electric convector heater, which is much safer.

Q My mother told me that it is very dangerous to give some kinds of foods to toddlers because it's possible they may choke on them. Is this true?

A Yes. Because they have not learned to chew properly, you do have to take care what you give to a child who is under three, especially if they are unsupervised for any length of time.

Never give hard sweets, pieces of apple, or any food in large chunks that could be difficult to swallow, and possibly cause an obstruction. Peanuts are the most dangerous of all, because there is a high risk that they will be swallowed whole. If this happens and a peanut gets lodged in the child's windpipe, turn him or her upside down and slap the back to dislodge it. If a peanut has reached the lungs, get the child to hospital as soon as possible. If the child's breathing stops, it is crucial to give mouth-to-mouth artificial respiration immediately.

Q When she has a temper tantrum, my little girl holds her breath until she goes blue in the face. Could she suffocate by doing this?

A No, because eventually the mechanisms of the body come into operation to start her breathing again—although this may not happen until she has lost consciousness for a few seconds. To stop the attack before it reaches this stage, try hooking your index finger over her tongue and pulling the tongue forward. This will make her take a breath.

Everyone should know how to give artificial respiration because it could save a life in an emergency.

Artificial respiration is the most important first aid technique for the relief of asphyxia. Asphyxia literally means 'absence of pulse', but is used to describe suffocation. A person who is suffocating is suffering from a lack of oxygen, which is normally obtained from breathing in the air. The victim struggles for breath and if this fight is unsuccessful, unconsciousness follows.

Causes of asphyxia

Oxygen is essential to keep the body alive and working and is carried to all parts via the bloodstream; a deficiency can have many causes. Air may not be able to get in and out of the nose and mouth because they are covered by a plastic bag, a pillow, or some other obstruction such as a sleeping cat in a baby's cot or pram. Or the airway between mouth and lungs may be blocked by food that has gone down the 'wrong way', a toy, the victim's tongue, broken or false teeth, or vomit. The airway can also be closed through swelling caused by swallowing scalding or corrosive liquid, or by an insect sting.

Any constriction of the neck, as in strangulation, has the same result. Sometimes the windpipe closes up naturally; this could happen because of noxious gases or through diseases such as bronchitis and asthma. Crushing of the chest, a common injury in car and crowd accidents, is another way in which the airway can be blocked.

Methods of artificial respiration

In the 'kiss of life', you take a deep breath, and after firmly sealing your lips over those of the victim, breathe out firmly.

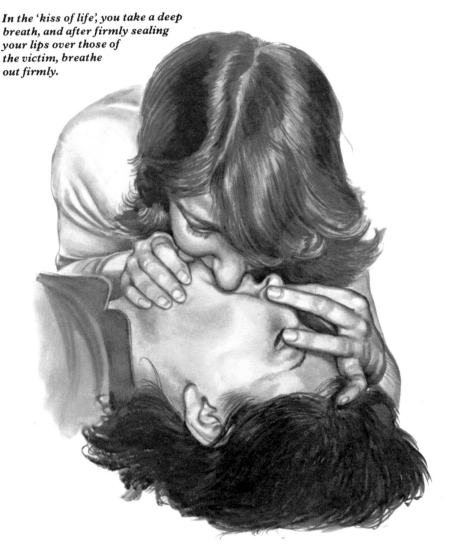

Even if the airway is clear, the body may still become deprived of oxygen. The air breathed in may contain carbon monoxide which will be absorbed by the tissues in place of oxygen. Cyanide (prussic acid) fumes can render the body incapable of using oxygen. Air full of smoke, gas or dust is low in oxygen and, if breathed in, can result in asphyxia.

The air at high altitude is 'thin' in oxygen and has the same effect. Respiration will also stop, bringing on asphyxia, if the nerves that control breathing are injured by electrocution, pesticides, excessive use of drugs such as morphia or barbiturates, or by the spinal cord being crushed.

Effects of asphyxia

Whatever its cause, the outcome of this lack of oxygen is the same. Breathing becomes deeper and more rapid as the body tries to compensate for the oxygen deficiency. At the same time, the heartbeat—and the pulse—speed up as the body desperately tries to get more oxygen to the tissues.

As the blood's oxygen content goes down, its carbon dioxide content rises and it turns from bright red to a bluish-purple. This change is reflected in the skin which turns blue, particularly in the face, neck and at the extremities (the hands and feet).

As the blood is increasingly deprived of oxygen, the brain ceases to function fully and the victim loses consciousness. When this happens, the brain may 'misfire', causing fits and foaming at the mouth. Finally, respiration will fail and soon afterwards the heart follows.

Life-saving action

Asphyxia is an emergency that demands drastic life-saving measures. Artificial respiration is most important as it not only gets breathing started again, but also increases the oxygen in the blood, which helps prevent permanent injury to the brain. The brain will suffer irreversible damage if it is totally starved of oxygen for a period lasting more than about four minutes.

Everyone should know how to give artificial respiration—when an accident occurs there is no time to look up the instructions in a book. But do not rush in and start artificial respiration without thinking first. If a room is filled with carbon monoxide or some other poisonous gas, it is essential to open the doors or windows first; if not, you too will soon be asphyxiated. In the case of electrocution it is vital to switch off the current before touching the victim. Should the asphyxia be caused by choking, try to dislodge any deep obstruction immediately.

Methods of artificial respiration

Mouth-to-mouth artificial respiration for an adult

You must be quick but careful. Learn this routine by heart in case you have to use it in an emergency when there is neither time nor opportunity to look up instructions in a book. Always make sure that clothing is loosened and the airway is clear before starting artificial respiration, but do not bother to try to drain the water from the lungs of someone who has drowned—this is a waste of precious time as there is no chance of removing the water completely. Points to remember during mouth to mouth resuscitation are to watch the victim's chest as you breathe into the lungs to make sure they are filling with air and to look for a fall in the chest as you take your mouth away. For maximum effect give the first five breaths as quickly as possible then aim for a rhythm of one breath every five seconds. Between breaths call for help if you are alone. If feasible try to pull the victim towards a window between breaths to get fresh air. Ask any onlookers to loosen any other tight clothing and to cover the victim with a coat or blanket. Most important of all, keep going.

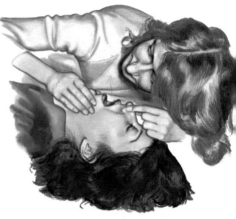

Put one hand under the chin and the other on the forehead so that your finger and thumb can reach the nose. Send any onlooker for help.

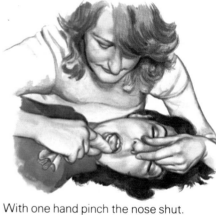

With one hand pinch the nose shut. Check the airway and remove any obstructions such as food, vomit or dentures by sweeping one finger round the mouth.

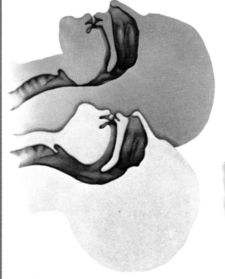

Turn the victim on his or her back and tilt the head back as far as possible so that the tongue falls against the palate and the airway is clear. Very quickly loosen any tight clothing at neck or waist.

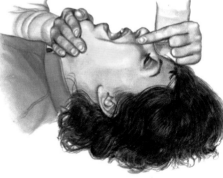

Administer the 'kiss of life' (see previous page). Now take your mouth away and watch the chest sink. Breathe in again and give five breaths quickly.

FIRST AID

Mouth-to-mouth artificial respiration for a baby or child.

The rules for giving mouth-to-mouth artificial respiration to a child are exactly as for an adult but it is important not to breathe out too hard as this may over-inflate the lungs.

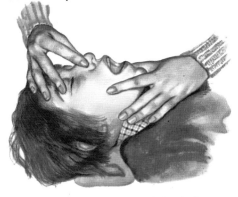

Clear the airway as for an adult, pinch the nose and take a shallow breath.

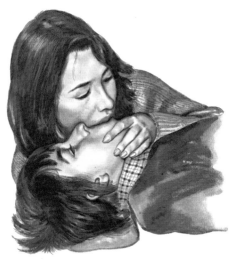

Breathe out very gently. For a very small child breathe into the nose and mouth.

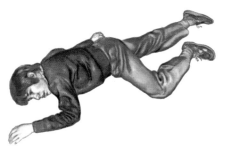

If the child starts to breathe, place him or her in the recovery position as shown.

The Silvester method

The Silvester method of artificial respiration should be used only as an alternative to the mouth-to-mouth method when an accident victim has facial injuries which make it impossible to place your mouth over the victim's, or because strong poison has been swallowed which could affect you as well, or if there is profuse vomiting, in which case the mouth-to-mouth method could cause choking by pushing vomit into the bronchial tubes and lungs. When using this method make sure that the support is under the victim's shoulders, not beneath the neck, so that the head can be bent back as far as possible for maximum clearance of the airway. As you press down on the victim's chest, make sure that you press on the lungs, not on the abdomen, which could damage internal organs. For a child press lightly to avoid internal damage.

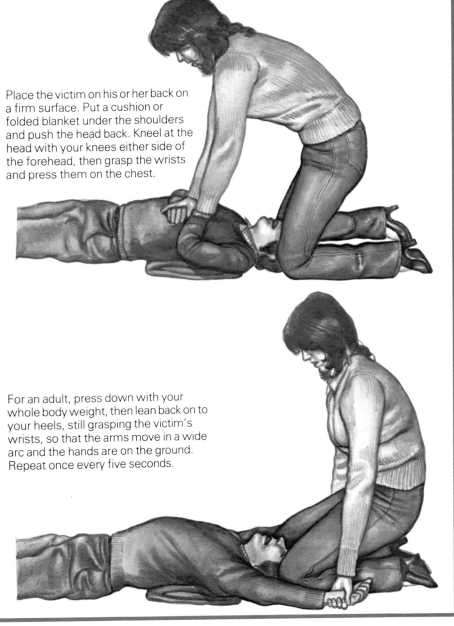

Place the victim on his or her back on a firm surface. Put a cushion or folded blanket under the shoulders and push the head back. Kneel at the head with your knees either side of the forehead, then grasp the wrists and press them on the chest.

For an adult, press down with your whole body weight, then lean back on to your heels, still grasping the victim's wrists, so that the arms move in a wide arc and the hands are on the ground. Repeat once every five seconds.

Hayward Art Group

Protecting your child from suffocation: some common hazards to avoid

Age	Risk	Preventive action
Birth to one year	**Choking**—on milk that is 'brought back'	Lie baby on front or side, not back. Never leave alone, feeding from propped-up bottle
	swallowing small object	Keep beads, buttons, marbles out of reach. Ensure soft toys have 'safety' eyes
	Suffocation—pillow falling on face	Do not give baby a pillow. Do not sleep with baby in your bed. If propping up child, put pillow under mattress
	plastic sticking to face	Cover plastic-lined pram or cot sides with loosely-woven cotton fabric e.g. muslin. Remove plastic cover from mattress. Keep spare plastic pants out of reach
One year upwards	cat going to sleep on baby's face	Do not keep cat, alternatively fit cat net on cot and pram
	Suffocation—plastic bag on head	Keep polythene bags out of reach. Knot ends of bag
	child climbing into old refrigerator	Remove door or use chain and padlock—better still, get refuse department to remove
	gas turned on	Fit fire-guard, have self-igniting type
	Drowning	Never leave toddler alone in bath; water must be shallow enough for child to be able to raise head when lying face down
		Cover ponds with wire mesh—better still fill in. Empty paddling pools after use
		Accompany child whenever paddling. Do not allow near rivers, lakes etc. without adults accompanying. Teach to swim as early as possible
	Electric shock	Be firm about not touching plugs
		Use safety plugs with shuttered sockets. Fit dummy plugs on unused sockets
		Do not give child electric blanket
		Check all appliances for wiring and earthing
		Avoid toys that are powered from mains

For an adult, quickly roll the victim on to his or her side and give several short, sharp slaps between the shoulder blades. For a child, turn upside down and slap on the back. Do not bother to try tipping the water from someone who has drowned—start artificial respiration immediately. Always use the 'kiss of life' or mouth-to-mouth method unless the victim has severe facial injuries (in which case use the Silvester method, as illustrated).

Points to remember

Always give the first five breaths as quickly as possible, to get a surge of oxygen into the blood and help prevent irreversible brain damage.

Do not blow too hard or the lungs may be damaged and air may get into the stomach, possibly causing vomiting.

If efforts seem to be useless because the airway from the mouth is completely blocked, try blowing air in through the victim's nose.

Keep a close watch on the heart. If it stops beating, get someone to start heart massage at 60 pressures a minute, or intersperse 15 pressures on the heart with two quick mouth-to-mouth breaths.

Most important of all, keep going—someone's life may depend on it.

Even against seemingly insuperable odds, the victim will usually respond to artificial respiration and start to breathe. When this starts it may be shallow, or breaths may come in intermittent gasps.

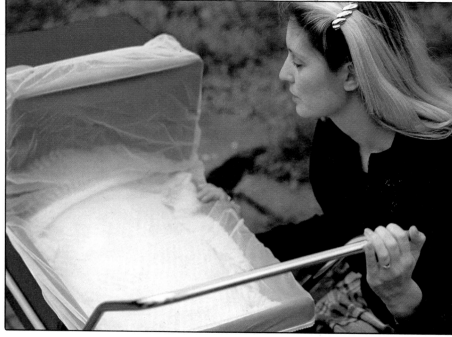

A net on the baby's pram deters cats from entering it and lying on the child, causing suffocation.

Stop to allow the patient a chance to breathe on his or her own, but if breathing is spasmodic give an extra small breath or two to help restore the normal breathing pattern.

Once the patient is breathing properly, turn him or her on to one side into the recovery position with the leg and arm bent; the other side of the body should be straight with the head facing towards the bent arm. The chin should tilt down so that any vomit can easily drain from the mouth. Unless it has been impossible to call for help until now, do not leave the victim on any account until emergency help arrives on the scene.

Asbestosis

Research shows that asbestos can cause severe lung disease. As a result, those working with it are protected by strict regulations and regular medical checks.

Asbestosis is the name given to the lung disease caused by the mineral asbestos. It most commonly affects people who, in the course of their work, have to handle the substance and are unable to avoid breathing in its microscopic fibres from the air.

Asbestos is an unusual mineral because it is naturally fibrous. It has proved useful for years because the fibres, after being extracted from the ore after mining, can be woven or compressed into a material that is heat-and fire-resistant. This makes it invaluable in the manufacture of textiles, for brake and clutch linings, and in the building industry, for boarding, piping, insulation, use in paints and as tiles.

The disease

Since asbestos was first used commercially towards the end of the 19th century, its ill effects have been noted. It only affects those people who work with the mineral which, when inhaled can cause fibrosis of the lungs (thickening of lung tissues). Minor forms of the disease are only detectable through chest X-rays.

Symptoms of asbestosis include a noticeable shortening of breath, a lack of oxygen in the blood that leads to the familiar 'blueness' known as cyanosis and the thickening of the ends of the fingers, called 'clubbing'.

Unfortunately, asbestos fibres can also cause cancer; they are able to penetrate the cells of the body, which can ultimately lead to cancer developing. Those directly related to asbestos exposure which affect the lining membrane of the lung or abdomen are lung cancer and cancers of the stomach and bowel.

This lung cancer is the same type as is caused by smoking, and asbestos workers who smoke are especially vulnerable.

The tumours are particularly related to exposure to blue asbestos, of which there is still a lot in lagging and buildings. So care has to be taken when replacing it or in demolition work.

Evidence concerning cancer of the bowel is less conclusive, but it would appear that workers who face contamination are certainly at risk.

Prevention

Ignorance about the effects of asbestos has caused great suffering in the past. In fact, tumours are still occurring that can be traced back to contamination 30 to 40 years ago.

Nowadays, the dangers are recognized and workers are protected by law. Strict regulations are laid down about working conditions, the provision of protective clothing and the wearing of masks, the monitoring of levels of asbestos in the air, and facilities for washing and showering.

Workers who deal with asbestos wear protective clothing and masks.

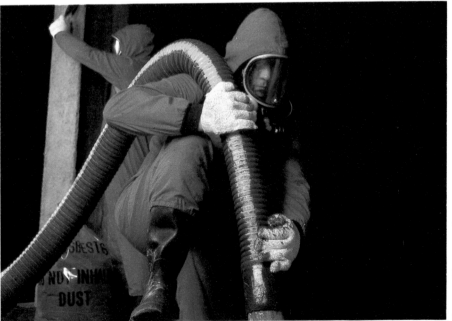

Courtesy of Envirocor Ltd

Aspirin and analgesics

Q Do painkillers act as sleeping tablets?

A Strictly speaking, no. Milder painkillers may help by relieving pain which has been disrupting sleep. Some of the stronger ones obtainable on prescription do also act as sedatives and can induce sleep.

Q I am taking an analgesic. Is it safe for me to drink alcohol?

A If you're using a mild analgesic— aspirin or paracetamol, say— there should be no problem in taking an occasional drink. However, both aspirin and undiluted spirits can cause bleeding in the gut, so it is wise to avoid the combination if you have a delicate stomach.

Alcohol is a good standby for severe pain, but it should never be taken at the same time as a strong painkiller because both substances slow down breathing, and the interaction of the two substances could be dangerous.

Q My husband gets bad migraines; if he doesn't get treatment straight away it always takes a long time for them to go. Why is this?

A What happens is that when a migraine attack occurs, the body shuts down the stomach. Once this happens, there is little chance of any drug being absorbed—so make sure your husband gets treatment immediately or his chances of a rapid recovery will be reduced. If this is impossible for any reason, your doctor may prescribe an analgesic in suppository form, or administer a drug orally that will assist absorption.

Q Can aspirin work as a male contraceptive pill?

A This is not as unlikely as it sounds, but the doses must be very large. Aspirin inhibits the production of prostaglandins, which are associated with sperm production. In an American study of analgesic abuse, few men became fathers while taking large doses of aspirin. But in animal tests, large doses caused their testicles to shrink and inhibited sperm production. Obviously, aspirin is an unreliable contraceptive.

There are many analgesics—or painkillers—easily available today, of which aspirin is the most widely advertised, but it is important to know the right analgesic to take to relieve a particular pain.

The range of pain-killing drugs available today can be confusing. Some are fairly mild, some are dangerous; many can be bought at the chemist's or supermarket, others obtained only on prescription.

The commonest analgesic is aspirin. It is used for ailments ranging from flu to fevers, from period pains to rheumatism, and is also, of course, the much heralded standby for 'tension headache'.

However, aspirin is not suitable for pain connected with the heart, gut or urinary tract, or for those who may develop rashes and breathing difficulties with it. Neither would paracetamol, another popular analgesic, be good for some people with liver trouble. If in any doubt, ask your chemist to recommend a suitable product. If pain persists, don't just take more tablets; see your doctor.

Painkillers in action

Pain is transmitted (A) by prostaglandins across synapses (gaps between a nerve ending and a new nerve beginning), along the nerves, and finally to the brain. Painkillers act (B) by inhibiting the production of prostaglandins.

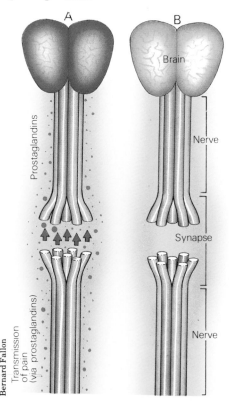

Bernard Fallon

Dosage
As a general rule, take a painkiller before pain really gets bad; use enough for it to work, but don't go over the suggested dose. With aspirin, this is 4gm, or 12 tablets, in 24 hours, or double that for acute rheumatism. For a two-year-old, the maximum is 150mg up to three times in 24 hours. Infants under a year should not have aspirin.

Types
Analgesics fall into one of two categories—those that act locally on a specific pain, and those that act centrally, from within, and which affect the whole nervous system.

The first group, known as peripheral painkillers, include aspirin, paracetamol and the once-popular phenacetin—now no longer used because of its effect on the kidneys. All these are used to relieve mild to moderate pain in muscles, joints or bones, and they work by reducing the body's production of substances called prostaglandins which cause muscles to contract, so making the person more susceptible to pain.

The centrally-acting painkillers are much more powerful and are therefore more strictly controlled by law. This category includes codeine, DF118 and distalgesic. It also covers all the opiates, whether natural or synthetic, and includes morphine and heroin as well as opium itself.

Opiates work by dulling pain through interacting with the brain's own naturally produced morphine-like substances called endorphins. They are all inclined to produce side-effects such as slow breathing, nausea, vomiting, constipation and—most serious of all—tolerance and addiction.

Codeine is also an opiate, but because it is relatively harmless, you can obtain it without prescription.

Alternatives
It is also worth noting that analgesics are not the only way to relieve pain. Non-chemical methods such as applying cold water (for burns and bruises) or heat and massage (for aches) can bring relief, while techniques on the fringes of orthodox medicine such as acupuncture, electrical stimulation, meditation and biofeedback are well worth trying in really chronic cases.

Painkillers—their uses and effects

Drug	Used for	Effects
Aspirin	Acute or chronic aches and pains (e.g. tension headache, period pains, neuralgia, toothache); flu; fevers; rheumatism	Fast-acting; reduces fever and inflammation; does not cause dependence in users. Can irritate stomach, affect hearing and cause rashes and breathing problems in some people
Paracetamol	Aches and pains; flu; fevers	Reduces fever; no gastric irritation. Does not reduce inflammation. Effects less prolonged than aspirin. Constant use can affect liver function
Codeine	Aches and pains; coughs; mild diarrhoea	Slightly constipating; in large doses can slow down breathing and cause nausea
Phenylbutazone	Rheumatic and joint disorders	Reduces inflammation and swelling. Can cause fluid retention, nausea and blood disorders
Morphine	Diarrhoea (with kaolin as liquid mixture); severe pain (e.g. in injuries, heart attack, coronary thrombosis, after surgery)	Swift and effective. Can cause constipation, nausea, slow breathing. Derived from opium and therefore addictive

DOs and DON'Ts of pain relief

DO
● take a painkiller soon after the pain begins, otherwise it will be more difficult to relieve it.
● find out how painkillers interact with any other medicines being taken.
● take painkillers with food or milk to reduce the risk of stomach irritation.
● give children smaller doses, as indicated on the label. If in doubt, ask the chemist about the correct dosage. Soluble painkillers are best for children; mix them in fruit juice or milk.
● buy medicines in childproof bottles and keep all drugs out of their reach
● induce vomiting if you suspect an overdose. Drinking salty water or thrusting two fingers down the throat usually brings it on.

DON'T
● take painkillers often or in large doses without medical advice.
● take more than the stated dose
● store painkillers, especially aspirin, in the bathroom or anywhere moist—they will perish. A cool, dry place is best.

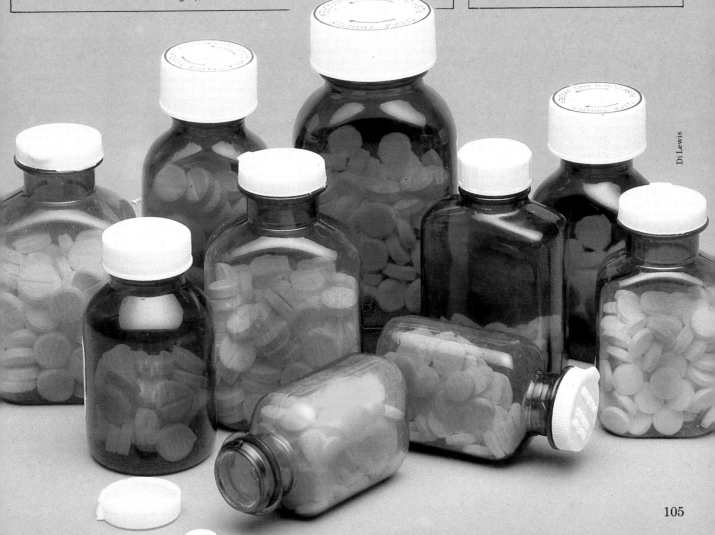

Di Lewis

Asthma

Q Is there anything I can do if I forget my inhaler and then suffer an attack?

A There is very little you can do and this sort of situation only serves to emphasize how important it is to carry your medication with you always. If you suffer a severe attack then you must go to a doctor or a hospital emergency department as soon as possible. In the meantime it is most important that you sit still and save your breath.

Q My father had asthma when he was a lad and my son and I have it. Can asthma run in families?

A Unfortunately, asthma does have a tendency to run in families, especially those asthmas which are a strong response to an allergy. The inherited link is not yet fully understood.

Q I use an inhaler for my asthma about five or six times a day. But I've heard that the inhaler is dangerous for the heart. Is this true?

A No. Bronchodilator inhalers had a bad reputation some years ago because they over-stimulated the heart. Modern inhalers affect the heart much less and so are far safer.

Q My two young children are both asthmatic, but they are also full of energy. Should they be allowed to play sports?

A Definitely yes. Any asthmatic should be vigorously encouraged to participate in sport. Some sports may be more likely to cause asthma than others, and in this case the child should make sure that he has his inhaler handy. Of all sports, swimming is the least likely to bring on an attack.

Q Why does my son always seem to get an asthmatic attack when we have guests?

A There is often a connection between emotional stress and asthma attacks. Try to make your son feel more relaxed. Involve him in the preparations, and avoid pushing him into the limelight.

Asthma is a very common respiratory complaint—so it is essential to know the symptoms, the treatments available, and the ways of preventing an attack.

Asthma involves a severe narrowing of the bronchial tubes. These lead from the windpipe—called the trachea—into the lungs and they carry the oxygen we breathe in to all parts of the lungs and provide a path for the carbon dioxide (a waste product of the body) to escape up the trachea when we breathe out.

The narrowing of the bronchial tubes—or bronchi—results from the contraction of the muscle lining them and causes difficulty in breathing that is most marked when breathing out. For this reason, asthmatics tend to breathe in in short gasps and breathe out with a long wheeze—a result of the effort required to breathe against the obstruction.

The body's defences

Two different chemicals are responsible for causing the bronchial muscles to contract. One is histamine, which is released from mast cells (cells that store histamine) as part of an allergic reaction and the other is acetyl choline which is a chemical released from the nerve endings which control the bronchial muscle.

These nerves are branches of the important vagus nerve which originates in the brain. The vagus keeps the bronchi in a constant state of contraction all the time and, as such, can be regarded as the main control over bronchial contraction, with additional control being provided by histamine.

To keep the balance between contraction and expansion (dilation), there are other substances that cause the bronchi to relax, thus working against the histamine and acetylcholine. These substances are called bronchodilators and a number of them are manufactured in the adrenal glands situated above each kidney.

The most important bronchodilator is adrenalin, which acts as a stimulant during periods of stress and excitement; when we need more oxygen to provide energy during a dangerous situation, the adrenalin helps to open up the bronchi to allow more air through to the lungs during rapid breathing.

In addition to this, the bronchial muscles also contain enzymes— substances which are responsible for maintaining certain bodily functions on which life depends; among these is respiration (breathing)—and these help to protect them from the action of histamine and acetyl choline.

The use of an inhaler containing a drug such as ventolin gives almost immediate relief from an asthmatic attack.

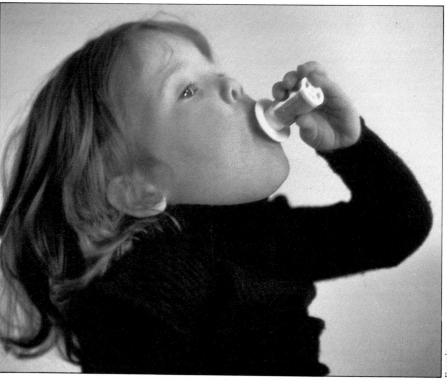

Fyson's

The respiratory system

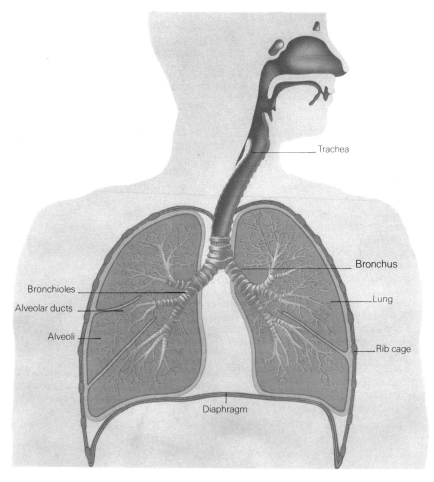

Trachea

Bronchus

Lung

Bronchioles

Alveolar ducts

Alveoli

Rib cage

Diaphragm

Causes

Asthma is brought on by a number of different causes, ranging from breathing polluted air to emotional upset, which makes it a rather complex problem to treat. However, since all the causes of asthma trigger the release of either histamine or acetyl choline, it is important to understand these two chemical reactions in order to see why people are vulnerable to asthma.

Histamine release is the most common cause of asthma, and the process which brings it about is rather remarkable considering that the substances which trigger it—house dust containing house mites, animal fur, pollen and fungal spores among others—are so varied.

Some people develop an excessive amount of an antibody (a protein made by the body as part of its defence system) to some substances breathed in—these substances (some of which are listed above) are known as allergens and they cause allergic reactions. It is this malfunction of the body's defences which starts the reaction leading to asthma.

What happens is that the antibody, which is known as immunoglobulin E, or IgE, attaches itself to the mast cells where the histamine is stored. The next time the allergen is inhaled, each molecule (particles which make up the whole antibody) of IgE pairs up with a neighbouring molecule and, as a result of this mating, the mast cell releases its store of histamine. The bronchi then begins to contract, making it increasingly difficult to breathe: the condition that we call asthma.

Acetyl choline released from the nerve endings in the bronchial tubes can be caused by a number of substances which irritate both the bronchial tubes and the nerve endings. These nerve endings then send messages to the vagus with the information that they have been irritated. In response, the vagus nerve then contracts the bronchial muscles and so starts asthmatic breathing difficulties. The same sort of irritation is caused by viral or bacterial infections of the throat, which explains why asthma tends to get worse with chest infections and colds.

We also know that emotional upsets or anxiety may occasionally worsen an asthmatic condition, though how this happens is not clear.

Unknown causes

Unfortunately, there are a number of causes of asthma which are not fully understood. For certain people, asthma frequently occurs after vigorous exercise, especially running. It is probable that both histamine and the vagus nerve are involved, though, generally speaking, the more vigorous the running and the cooler the air which is breathed, the worse the asthma becomes.

Certain drinks, foods and preservatives can also produce an asthmatic response. Rather than being a straightforward allergic response, it is often the result of the body's sensitivity to certain substances. Again, the mechanism involved is still not fully understood.

Symptoms

The typical asthma attack is characterized by a sudden shortness of breath and wheezing, which is sometimes accompanied by coughing. The bringing up of phlegm is not a prominent part of the attack and suggests that the patient may also have bronchitis. Generally speaking, asthmatics are more prone to chest infections, and this is caused by a failure to clear the lungs fully. Many patients often develop a hunched look which is brought about by the constant effort of breathing.

In many cases, the onset of asthma follows a seasonal pattern as the pollen count rises. This pattern is often accompanied by irritations to the nose and sneezing, which we usually refer to as hay fever.

Of course, allergies to house pets and the house mite will occur all through the year as the allergen is constantly in the

The microscopic house mite, present in dust and bedding, can trigger an attack.

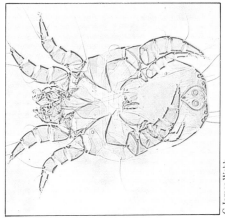

C James Webb

Asthma: its causes and prevention

Although an asthmatic condition must always be treated with drugs and according to the doctor's advice, there are some preventive measures that can be taken.

Causes	Preventive measures
INFECTIONS: common cold, some viral infections, sinusitis, bronchitis	Avoid groups and individuals with colds; stick to balanced diet, have adequate sleep, take moderate exercise
ALLERGENS BREATHED IN: pollens, house dust, feathers, fungal spores, animal hair	Keep house as dust-free as possible. Use foam pillows; avoid animals; fit electronic air cleaners
IRRITANTS BREATHED IN: fumes, like tobacco smoke, paint fumes; air pollutants; cold air	Avoid all fumes; stop smoking and avoid smokers; avoid going out into cold air
FOOD ALLERGENS: Can include milk, eggs, strawberries, fish, tomatoes	Isolate allergen through prick test and then avoid it
PSYCHOLOGICAL CHANGES: stress, emotional disturbance	Reduce or eliminate causes of stress; stop worrying, and avoid emotional disturbance
TRIGGER MECHANISMS: physical exertion; sudden changes in temperature	Avoid sudden physical exertion; approach exercise in relaxed manner; avoid constant temperature changes
DRUGS: Can include penicillin, vaccines, anaesthetics	Identify drugs that cause allergic reaction and avoid them. There are alternatives available

air. The house mite is particularly keen on living in warm places, like beds, and for this reason asthma attacks often seem to happen at night. In fact, coughing at night in children may well be a result of this allergy.

Treatment

The treatment given for asthma largely depends on the type of asthma and the severity of the attacks, but it is broadly divided into two: emergency treatment for severe attacks, requiring a visit from the doctor or admission to hospital, and everyday self-medication to prevent an attack occurring, which is known as prophylactic, or preventive, treatment and can be carried out at home.

The aim of emergency treatment is to bring relief as rapidly as possible and so one of three drugs is given by injection: adrenalin, aminophylline and hydro-cortisone, and these have an almost instantaneous effect. The first two act directly on the bronchial muscles, raising the enzyme level and so relaxing the muscle. The third is a steriod, and although it acts quickly to relieve the attack, how it works is not known. In very severe cases, oxygen may also be given to the patient.

Most asthmatics take some form of daily treatment, usually in the form of tablets or inhalers. The doctor will decide which type of drug is the most suitable after first diagnosing the cause of the asthma. To do this the prick test is used. This determines whether the asthma is a result of an allergic reaction and what the body is allergic to. A number of possible

allergens are introduced into the body through the skin. If the body reacts to any of these and produces a red weal, then the person is allergic to that particular allergen. A doctor may also measure the patient's breathing rate and capacity using a flow meter. This indicates just how much he or she is affected by the allergen.

Once the doctor has identified the most likely cause of the asthma he will prescribe the appropriate treatment. Wherever possible the allergen should be avoided. Drugs like intal – taken by inhalation – may be prescribed to decrease the release of histamine. Or a broncho-dilator, such as ventolin, taken either as

tablets or inhaled will give rapid relief from the effects of a sudden asthma attack, though not all people will react to the drug with the same speed.

For those who suffer from a more persistent and severe form of asthma, doctors may prescribe steroid drugs. Because of the side-effects of this type of drug, patients will be asked to stick rigidly to the doctor's recommended dosage, and to make sure that they always have the drug with them in case of an attack. The treatment should always be continued, as failure to do this may encourage a further attack.

Prevention and outlook

Most asthmatics will have their condition worsened or even triggered by everyday substances, and once the cause is identified, the only course is to avoid it by, for instance, keeping the house as clear of dust as possible, avoiding petrol fumes and tobacco smoke, and also sudden exertion and emotional stress. There are, of course, many other irritants, but these are the more common ones that can worsen an asthmatic condition.

However, it is difficult to be specific as what affects one asthmatic may actually have a beneficial effect on another. But it is accepted that regular, controlled exercise rather than sudden exertion does have a beneficial effect, and all asthmatics should be encouraged to take as much regular – but strictly controlled – exercise as they can manage at any one time.

Although there is no absolute cure – 50 per cent of child sufferers tend to grow out of the complaint during adolescence – asthmatics should be encouraged by the news that current research is producing positive results.

How histamine causes asthma

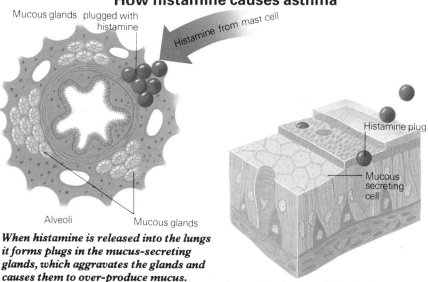

Mucous glands plugged with histamine

Histamine from mast cell

Alveoli

Mucous glands

Histamine plug

Mucous secreting cell

Section through alveolar tissue

When histamine is released into the lungs it forms plugs in the mucus-secreting glands, which aggravates the glands and causes them to over-produce mucus.

Venner Artists

Astigmatism

Q I have noticed that my son often squints and narrows his eyes almost to a slit when he is watching television. Do you think it is possible that he might have an astigmatism?

A This is quite possible. Screwing the eyes up like this—which is simply a way of compensating for the distortion caused by astigmatism—is in fact one of the commonest signs used in the diagnosis of the condition.

You should take your son to the optician to have his eyes tested regularly. Astigmatism can be corrected satisfactorily with glasses. Do not delay, because poor sight may affect the child's progress at school.

Q For years now I have been wearing fairly strong glasses because I have an astigmatism and am also very short-sighted. But I like the idea of wearing contact lenses. Will this be possible with my eye condition?

A You would probably be able to wear hard contact lenses. These work by taking over the function of the cornea. Even severe astigmatism and 'irregular' corneal astigmatism can be corrected with the wearing of hard lenses.

The only kind of soft contact lenses which would be suitable for your astigmatism are those of a 'toric' design, which do not rotate on the eye and may be slightly thicker at the bottom. But even this kind of lens is not always satisfactory.

Q I suffer from astigmatism and am wondering if my children are at all likely to inherit the same problem.

A It is possible. For instance, if the rare condition of albinism—an absence of pigment that causes skin and hair to be white and the eyes to be unable to bear normal light or focus properly—exists in your family, you should consult your doctor as to the probability of your children inheriting the condition.

However, if your own astigmatism was caused by surgery or an injury, then your children will most certainly not inherit it.

Astigmatism is an eye condition which can cause blurred vision, headaches and fatigue. However, the right glasses or contact lenses can usually correct the problem.

If the curve of the front surface of the cornea, the outer covering of the eye, is irregular, the person will see a distorted image. This particular kind of sight defect is called astigmatism.

In fact, nearly everyone's eyes are affected to some extent by astigmatism, because very rarely does the front surface of the cornea provide a perfect lens. If the irregularity is slight, vision will not be noticeably affected. If it is marked, however, the image will be distorted—with vertical, horizontal or diagonal blurring, depending on the nature of the imperfection—and the condition will require treatment.

Causes
Astigmatism may be present from birth or it may develop in childhood over a number of years. Severe astigmatism may be inherited. Sometimes it is secondary to other eye conditions or it can result from the formation of scar tissue after the cornea has been diseased or injured. Or it may follow eye operations such as the removal of cataracts.

Occasionally, distortion may be caused by a part of the eye other than the cornea. Even slight dislocation of the lens inside the eye—for example, from a severe blow—will produce a warped image. So

will disease or pressure behind the eye affecting the fovea, the pinhead-sized area of the retina used for acute vision. But it is the cornea which is responsible for most cases.

Diagnosis and treatment
Astigmatism should be suspected in someone who narrows his or her eyelids almost to a slit in order to see more clearly. Diagnosis requires careful assessment of the irregularities of the cornea, testing with special patterns to determine exactly which part of the image is distorted and how severely. Instruments used to measure astigmatism include the retinoscope, which allows the light reflections from the inside of the eye to be studied, and the keratometer, which measures the corneal images.

Astigmatism is harder to correct than straightforward long or short sight. The commonest way is to prescribe glasses with cylindrical lenses ground to the required curvature, though the wearer may still notice some blurring. If, as often happens, astigmatism is accompanied by short or long sight, compound spectacle lenses are the answer.

Contact lenses may also be used, and very severe cases of 'irregular' astigmatism may call for a corneal graft.

Comparison of normal and astigmatic sight

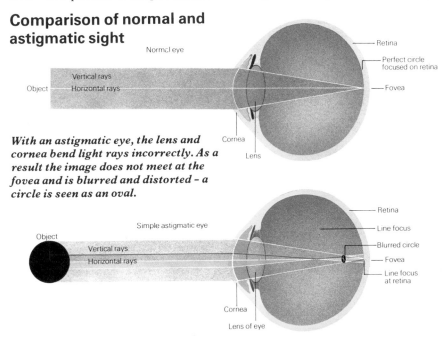

Normal eye

Object — Vertical rays — Horizontal rays

Cornea — Lens

Retina — Perfect circle focused on retina — Fovea

With an astigmatic eye, the lens and cornea bend light rays incorrectly. As a result the image does not meet at the fovea and is blurred and distorted – a circle is seen as an oval.

Simple astigmatic eye

Object — Vertical rays — Horizontal rays

Cornea — Lens of eye

Retina — Line focus — Blurred circle — Fovea — Line focus at retina

Hayward Art Group

Athlete's foot

Q I have a severe form of athlete's foot that keeps recurring. Is there any chance that the condition will leave my feet scarred or deformed?

A Thankfully, the fungus causing athlete's foot lives only on the superficial layers of the skin, eating dead skin cells. For this reason, there will be no scarring, but in chronic cases the nails may become affected and need specialist treatment with drugs. With correct treatment of skin and nails, the foot should return to normal.

Q I have grown weary of trying to get rid of athlete's foot. But every time I think it has gone for good, it makes a comeback. Is there a reason for this?

A The commonest reason for re-infection is that the fungus has never been properly eradicated in the first place. For this reason it is important to dust your shoes and socks, as well as your feet with antifungal powder as they can carry the fungus. It is also important to keep up the medical treatment for a considerable time after the symptoms have disappeared.

Q I have suffered from athlete's foot for some time now, and have just discovered a similar sort of irritation on my hands. Is it possible for athlete's foot to spread to other parts of the body?

A The athlete's foot fungus belongs to a group of fungi known as Trichophytons and these can live on various parts of the body. But they are not very contagious and so are unlikely to spread. However, there is a condition similar to athlete's foot that can affect the hands, and this should be diagnosed and treated by the doctor.

Q My daughter has athlete's foot. Can this spread to the rest of the family?

A Not if precautions are taken, the most important being hygiene; everyone should carefully wash and dry his or her own feet—with a personal towel—and use an antifungal powder on feet and shoes.

Athlete's foot is annoying and unpleasant, but usually responds well to treatment—and can be prevented.

Athlete's foot is a fungal infection and probably the most common foot complaint that doctors treat. It can affect almost everyone, though small children do appear to be immune.

Causes

The only real cause of athlete's foot is a failure to observe the necessary personal hygiene, along with carelessness in drying the feet after a bath. Those people who suffer from sweaty feet are particularly prone to this complaint and the situation can be aggravated by wearing airless, plastic shoes which prevent the feet from breathing.

It is the moist, sweaty areas between the toes that provide the soggy skin on which the fungus likes to settle. The fungus then lives on the skin, digesting the dead skin that the body sheds each day. Once the fungus starts eating the dead skin, it may then cause inflammation and damage to the living skin.

There is a small risk of picking up athlete's foot in bathrooms and in public changing rooms.

Symptoms and treatment

The first sign of athlete's foot is irritation and itching between the toes followed by the skin beginning to peel. This can be accompanied by bad foot odour.

In worse cases, painful red cracks, known as fissures, appear between the toes, and in the odd severe case, the toenails become affected. These become either soft or more brittle as the fungus invades the nail substance. It may be possible to see the nail thickening beneath its outer shell. In extreme cases, the foot swells and blisters—requiring prompt attention from the doctor.

Modern antifungal creams and powders are successful in the treatment of athlete's foot. Substances such as clotrimazole and tolnafate are extremely effective as creams or ointments, and need to be applied daily while the condition lasts, and for two or three weeks after the symptoms have disappeared to prevent its recurrence.

Where the infection is severe and the nails have been affected a drug known as griseofulvin may be prescribed by the doctor to be taken orally. It is effective within a few weeks. It is then necessary to dust the feet, socks and shoes with antifungal powder to prevent re-infection.

Athlete's foot can be treated at home, but if the problem begins to spread or refuses to respond to treatment then your doctor must be consulted.

Preventing athlete's foot
Chances of developing athlete's foot can be reduced by following a few guidelines on foot care.
* Wash the feet daily with soap, and clean all dirt from under the nails and between toes
* Dry each toe thoroughly with your own towel, paying particular attention to the gaps between toes
* Powder your feet with antifungal powder. To prevent re-infection also powder shoes
* Put on clean cotton or wool socks daily. Avoid nylon socks and plastic shoes. Wear open shoes if feet feel sweaty

The white, peeling skin of athlete's foot (left) can be treated with an antifungal powder (below). This can also be used to prevent infection where risk exists.

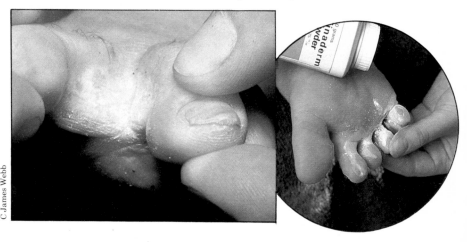

C James Webb

Attachment in infancy

Q My two-year-old son always clings to me whenever I take him to a children's party, though he is quite independent at home. Should I push him socially?

A Don't push him at all. In time, his confidence will increase and he will learn to cope with his shyness. Some children take quite a while to lose their reserve, and if you stay in the background at a party, you may eventually find there is a sudden burst of confidence.

Why not say at the beginning: 'Do you remember how much you enjoyed yourself last time? Well, I'll stay again this time, but if I see you are having a good time, I may slip out to do a bit of shopping; then I'll come back at the end.' This way, you should be able to leave without causing a disturbance and your child will be prepared.

Q I am going into hospital soon to have my second baby. Is there any way I can prepare my toddler for my absence?

A She is sure to miss you. And on your return you may find she either ignores you or becomes very demanding. All you can do is make sure things run smoothly while you are away and that she is looked after by someone she knows. Make sure it is someone you know and that she trusts. The more she becomes used to being handled by other people, the easier she will be able to cope with your absence.

Q In all the articles I read about attachment forming the emphasis is placed on the mother. Doesn't the father have a place? As an expectant 'dad', surely I can have as close a relationship with my baby as my wife?

A If this is what you want, then of course you can. Doctors seem to think that the baby forms the strongest attachment with the individual who looks after it most. So if you are going to share in the birth as much as you are able, and expect to share the responsibilities of your baby's everyday care, then it is likely that the bonding will be equally shared and you will be able to develop a close and loving relationship with your child.

It is important for a baby's emotional development that a loving attachment is formed with the mother – or whoever is to care for it – from birth. What, then, are the best ways of ensuring that this happens?

Babies have the ability to share a responsive and loving relationship from the moment they are born. But because of the way sexual roles are defined, a father may not be present at the birth, and the baby is first handed to the mother, making her the child's early contact.

Opinion is divided as to whether the strong bond that occurs between the mother and the infant is 'natural' or the result of conditioning from birth onwards. On the one hand, babies are said to respond more to the female voice, and that since it is women who are biologically equipped to bear children and breast-feed them, the bonding must be physiological. Others argue that attachment still occurs when a mother substitute takes over.

Bonding at birth

It is a common practice when a woman has given birth for the baby to be taken away, washed and wrapped in a blanket before being handed to the mother. Nowadays, some midwives are questioning this rather efficient, hygienic approach, and some hospitals are handing the newborn infant to the mother—often with the umbilical cord still attached – straight after the birth.

Medical evidence seems to suggest that this has important implications for the future and encourages the relationship between mother and baby.

Babies that experience early caressing, eye-to-eye contact, and the sound of their mother's voice in those few hours after the birth, appear to cry less, be more alert and responsive. Even later in their development, they appear to have a more relaxed relationship with their mothers and are more receptive, and their mothers more understanding.

Problems with bonding

Unfortunately, love is not something that you can turn on at will, and with some women the bonding can take longer to establish, or even prove absent altogether. The reasons for this are complex and varied, but can usually be traced back to the woman's own childhood and upbring-

Those moments after the birth are important for the baby and parents.

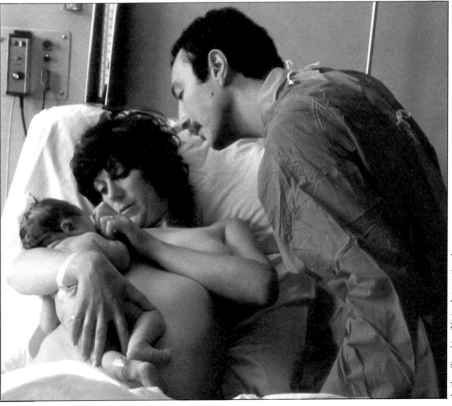

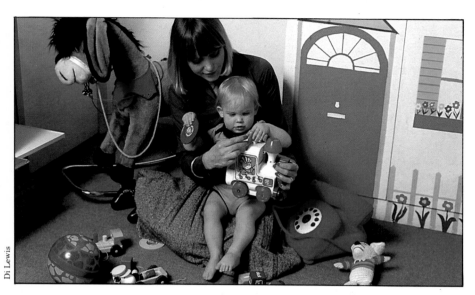

Di Lewis

ing. She may have been unloved and neglected; she may fear handling such a small creature because of her own insecurity; or the baby simply may not be as appealing and attractive as she had hoped. A woman can suffer great conflict and unhappiness if her ideal of motherhood does not match up with the reality.

Health visitors are trained to recognize the negative feelings that mothers may display and provide encouragement and support. They may be able to put an unhappy mother in touch with a local self-help group that offers support to women in a state of post-natal depression.

Making the adjustment

A woman who is at ease with herself is more likely to be at ease with her baby. It is this loving acceptance that enables children to grow up and mature into secure adults.

Learning how to cope with your own emotions is also a basis for good mothering. For example, if you feel rising panic at the sound of your baby crying, stop what you are doing, take a few deep breaths and you will find that you become more relaxed and listen with a less acute feeling of anxiety. Sometimes you may have negative feelings of your own: anger, coldness, a lack of interest. It can be very wearisome to feel that you always have to respond to your child's every demand. You will soon learn to identify your baby's cries so that you can distinguish between a cry of hunger, a shriek of pain, a yell of impatience, a whimper of loneliness and the restless cry of the simply bored.

Giving attention

When you give your attention to your baby, give it wholly. Talk continually; the words may be meaningless but children will respond to the tone.

A mother's close attention to her baby is essential to forming the early attachment so important for future development.

Not all the effort should be made by the mother, however. Babies respond just as happily to other adults, especially if they are used to them from the beginning. They are not only useful because they can lift some of the responsibility from the mother, but also because in forming a relationship with the baby they offer the beginnings of independence. Brothers and sisters can help in this way too.

Coping with clinging

All children cling to their mothers at some stage in their development. This usually happens between the ages of 18 months and three years. It takes the form of constant interruptions, creating a disturbance in a public place, and literally hanging on to mother's skirts.

This is an extremely trying stage, but there are two alternatives for solving the problems. First, you can give the attention as, when and where it is demanded, or you can give yourself a regular break by getting someone else to take over. Otherwise, find out where the nearest crèche is, to give your child the opportunity of being with other children of a similar age—and also give you a break.

Start the routine when the baby is under six months old, when it is more likely to adapt to new people.

Going back to work

Many mothers want to return to work when their babies are still small. Ideally, a good substitute mother should be provided, someone who will stay in your home and whose ideas on childrearing are similar to your own. Babies can adapt to substitute mothers without suffering

any obvious harm, and there is certainly no proof that children of working mothers grow up any less well adjusted than those of mothers who stay at home.

The moment of leaving a child is inevitably traumatic. The baby may initially cling or scream, causing the mother anguish and anxiety for the rest of the day. The best thing to do is to say goodbye firmly, with a confident smile and then to go without looking back and ignore any wails of outrage.

Usually children adjust quickly. But if the baby continues to cry, and after several days is still not adjusting and even showing signs of fear or of becoming withdrawn, you may have to rethink your plan. Perhaps you have chosen the wrong person or the wrong form of childcare; or perhaps a single incident has triggered off such a response. In this case, it is time for reassurance and a fresh start.

By the age of three, most children recognize the fact that other children and the outside world are more interesting and can provide as much fun as mother and father. They will go happily to playschool, though it may be wise to start this on a part-time basis. As they play with other children and learn from other adults, the ties will loosen. The bonding, in terms of love and affection will remain, with fewer strings attached.

Favourable factors

In hospital
● Holding the baby immediately after it is born
● Baby kept with mother; access at all times
● Breast-feeding (on demand, if required)
● Flexible visiting hours so father can be present as often as possible
● Good, sympathetic nursing; friendly, relaxed atmosphere
● Continual reassurance for mother and baby gained through cuddling, rocking, caressing

At home
● Good relationship between parents; loving, supportive father
● Continuing affection and reassurance
● Recognition of baby's individuality and need to develop resourcefulness
● Encouraging affection between baby and others, apart from parents
● Contact with other babies and children
● Ability of mother to 'let go', allowing baby to get to know other people and so develop independence